Table of Contents

20: Final Word

Introduction

Many people find it incredibly challenging to lose weight. With countless diets and weight loss programs available, it's easy to get overwhelmed and confused about which approach to take. As someone who has witnessed these struggles firsthand, I decided to write this comprehensive book, "Easy Weight Loss Diet for Maximum Results," to offer a practical and effective solution to this common problem.

The purpose of this book is simple: to help people achieve their weight loss goals in an easy, healthy, and secure manner. Through careful research, personal experience, and consultation with experts, I have devised a weight loss plan that is not only straightforward to follow but also ensures your well-being and safety throughout the journey.

The path to a healthier lifestyle should not be filled with frustrations and obstacles. That's why I advocate for an easy approach to weight loss. By simplifying the process, we can make it more accessible and attainable for everyone.

An easy weight loss approach involves making gradual, sustainable changes to your dietary habits and lifestyle. Instead of drastic measures that lead to quick fixes but often result in short-term gains, we will focus on long-term strategies that promote lasting results. By taking small steps and setting achievable goals, you can build a strong foundation for your weight loss journey.

Losing weight is not just about shedding pounds; it's about improving your overall health and well-being. Crash diets and extreme weight loss methods may provide rapid results, but they can also be detrimental to your body and mind. Opting for a healthy weight loss plan ensures that you nourish your body with the right nutrients and maintain an optimal balance.

The "Easy Weight Loss Diet for Maximum Results" emphasizes the importance of a balanced and nutritious diet. By incorporating a variety of fruits, vegetables, lean proteins, and whole grains, you can fuel your body with essential vitamins and minerals. We will also explore portion control and mindful eating techniques to help you develop a positive relationship with food.

Safety should be a top priority when it comes to weight loss. Unfortunately, the weight loss industry is saturated with fad diets, supplements, and products that promise quick results but may carry potential risks. In our journey towards a healthier lifestyle, we will prioritize security by avoiding any extreme or harmful practices.

This diet plan is rooted in science and supported by evidence-based approaches to weight loss. We will focus on natural, whole foods that provide essential nutrients and avoid any artificial additives or chemicals that might jeopardize your health. The goal is to create a safe and sustainable weight loss plan that you can confidently follow.

Gone are the days of dreading fasting or pushing yourself to the limits with intense physical exercises. This weight loss plan is designed to be adaptable to your everyday routine. You don't have to sacrifice your work, studies, or travel plans to achieve your weight loss goals.

The beauty of this approach lies in its integration with your daily activities. By making simple adjustments to your eating habits and incorporating light physical activities into your day, you can seamlessly incorporate weight loss efforts into your busy schedule. This way, you won't feel overwhelmed or burdened, increasing the chances of long-term success.

Another essential aspect of this weight loss plan is its inclusivity. It is formulated to cater to both men and women, recognizing the unique nutritional needs and preferences of each gender. Age, background, and fitness level should not be barriers to achieving a healthier lifestyle, and this diet plan ensures that everyone can participate.

By accommodating different dietary requirements and tastes, we aim to make this weight loss journey enjoyable and sustainable for all. Whether you're a working professional, a busy parent, a student, or a frequent traveler, this diet can be adapted to suit your individual circumstances.

In the following chapters of this book, I will guide you through the specifics of the "Easy Weight Loss Diet for Maximum Results." We will delve into the list of foods that are permitted and those to be avoided. I will share meal planning tips, delicious and nutritious recipes, and practical strategies to overcome common challenges in weight loss.

Remember that this book is not a quick fix. Instead, it offers a balanced and sensible approach to weight loss that prioritizes your well-being. With dedication and commitment, you can achieve maximum results and embark on a transformative journey towards a healthier, happier you.

Before making significant changes to your diet, especially if you have any underlying health conditions, it is essential to seek advice from a healthcare professional or a qualified nutritionist. Consulting with an expert will ensure that the modifications you plan to implement are safe and appropriate for your individual health needs. They can provide personalized guidance, taking into account your medical history, current health status, and dietary preferences, to help you make informed decisions that support your overall well-being. Remember that everyone's body is unique, and what works well for one person may not be suitable for another.

Prioritizing your health and seeking professional advice can lead to a more successful and sustainable approach to improving your diet and achieving your wellness goals.

The Key Principles of This Diet

In Chapter 1, we introduced the concept of the "Easy Weight Loss Diet for Maximum Results" and emphasized its focus on being easy, healthy, and secure. Now, in Chapter 2, we will delve deeper into the specific key principles and rules that form the foundation of this transformative diet plan. By understanding and implementing these essential guidelines, you can maximize your chances of success and achieve your weight loss goals in a sustainable and health-conscious manner.

One of the fundamental principles of this diet is the exclusion of added sugar. Sugar, especially in the form of refined sugars and high-fructose corn syrup, can be found in a wide range of foods, from sweet treats to processed snacks and even some seemingly "healthy" options. Consuming excessive amounts of sugar can lead to weight gain, fluctuating energy levels, and an increased risk of chronic health conditions.

To achieve the desired results from this weight loss plan, it is crucial to avoid any food that contains added sugar. This means cutting out sugary sodas, sugary snacks, candies, and sugary baked goods. Always check food labels for hidden sugars in processed foods and be mindful of ingredients like dextrose, sucrose, and other sweeteners.

By embracing a sugarless diet, you can stabilize your blood sugar levels, reduce cravings for sugary foods, and pave the way for healthier eating habits. In addition to sugar, salt can also be a significant contributor to weight gain and other health issues, such as high blood pressure and water retention. Therefore, this diet emphasizes reducing salt intake to promote better overall health and weight loss.

Avoid adding excessive amounts of salt while cooking, and be cautious of processed foods that are often high in sodium. Canned soups, packaged snacks, and fast food meals tend to contain excessive amounts of salt. Instead, opt for fresh ingredients and incorporate herbs and spices to enhance the flavor of your meals without relying on excess salt. By reducing salt intake, you may notice improvements in your body's water balance, leading to reduced bloating and a healthier, more balanced system.

Processed foods are often loaded with preservatives, artificial additives, and unhealthy fats, making them less nutritious and potentially harmful to your weight loss journey. As a crucial principle of this diet, it is essential to steer clear of processed foods altogether. Instead, focus on incorporating whole and natural foods into your daily meals. Whole foods are minimally processed or unprocessed, providing your body with essential nutrients and supporting healthy weight loss. Vegetables, fruits, whole grains, lean proteins, and nuts should form the foundation of your diet. By adopting this approach, you will be providing your body with the nutrients it needs to function optimally while reducing your overall calorie intake.

While the notion of "fat-free" may have been popularized in various weight loss trends, it's essential to understand the importance of healthy fats in a balanced diet. Not all fats are bad for you; in fact, some fats are crucial for maintaining overall health.

In this diet, we encourage the consumption of healthy fats in moderation while limiting the intake of saturated and trans fats. Healthy fats can be found in avocados, nuts, seeds, olive oil, and fatty fish such as salmon.

On the other hand, when it comes to dairy products and other food items, opt for low-fat or fat-free versions to reduce your overall calorie intake. Remember that moderation is key, and it's essential to strike a balance between healthy fats and controlling overall calorie intake to support your weight loss goals.

Fast food, junk food, and fried, greasy meals are notorious for their high-calorie content and lack of nutritional value. Consuming these types of foods regularly can sabotage your weight loss efforts and negatively impact your health.

As a rule of this diet, avoid fast food chains and opt for healthier, homemade alternatives. Replace greasy fried foods with healthier cooking methods such as baking, grilling, or steaming. Incorporate whole grains, lean proteins, and plenty of vegetables into your meals to make them more satisfying and nutrient-dense.

By cutting out fast food and junk food, you'll be eliminating empty calories and replacing them with nourishing options that will fuel your body and support your weight loss goals. While the key principles mentioned above form the backbone of this diet, it's essential to remember the importance of hydration and regular physical activity in achieving your weight loss goals.

Staying hydrated is crucial for overall health and can aid in weight loss. Water helps flush out toxins from your body, supports proper digestion, and can even help control your appetite. Make it a habit to drink plenty of water throughout the day and consider replacing sugary beverages with water or other low-calorie options.

Additionally, incorporating regular exercise into your daily routine can enhance your weight loss efforts. Exercise not only burns calories but also helps build lean muscle mass, which can increase your metabolism and support long-term weight management. Find physical activities that you enjoy, whether it's walking, dancing, cycling, or swimming, and aim to be active for at least 30 minutes most days of the week.

Alongside the specific dietary rules, portion control and mindful eating are essential aspects of this weight loss plan. Even when consuming healthy foods, overeating can hinder your progress towards your weight loss goals.

Practice portion control by being mindful of the serving sizes and avoid eating until you feel overly full. Eating slowly and savoring each bite can help you recognize feelings of fullness and prevent unnecessary overeating. Pay attention to hunger cues and emotions that may trigger eating, and try to distinguish between physical hunger and emotional cravings.

By incorporating portion control and mindful eating into your daily habits, you can better manage your calorie intake and create a healthy relationship with food.

As you embark on your weight loss journey with the "Easy Weight Loss Diet for Maximum Results," it's essential to track your progress and make adjustments as needed. Keep a food journal to record your meals, snacks, and beverages, along with any changes in your weight, energy levels, or mood.

By keeping track of your dietary habits, you can identify patterns and make informed decisions about what works best for you. Remember that everyone's body is different, and what may work for one person may not be the best approach for another. Listen to your body, and if you encounter challenges or plateaus, consider consulting with a healthcare professional or a registered dietitian to tailor the diet to your individual needs.

Embracing the key principles of the "Easy Weight Loss Diet for Maximum Results" is not just about losing weight; it's about fostering a healthier and more sustainable lifestyle. By prioritizing natural, whole foods, cutting out added sugars, reducing salt intake, and making smart fat choices, you will nourish your body and provide it with the essential nutrients it needs.

Avoiding fast food, junk food, and greasy meals will protect your body from empty calories and support your overall well-being. Coupled with hydration, regular exercise, portion control, and mindful eating, this diet becomes a powerful tool for achieving your weight loss goals while promoting overall health and vitality.

The Roadmap to Success

In order to achieve success in anything, one needs to invest time and effort, and losing weight is no exception. With the "Easy Weight Loss Diet for Maximum Results" and some positive lifestyle changes, attaining your weight loss goals is entirely within reach.

Determination plays a crucial role in your weight loss journey. Staying committed to your goals and reminding yourself of the reasons why you want to lose weight will help you stay focused and motivated.

This diet is designed to be sustainable, and it's essential to continue following it until you reach your desired results. Avoid falling into the trap of quick fixes or yo-yo dieting, and trust the process to bring about gradual but steady progress.

To monitor your progress, consider keeping a progress diary. Document your daily experiences, challenges, and successes, including meals, snacks, exercise routines, and how you feel both physically and emotionally. This journal will be a valuable resource to track your achievements, identify patterns, and make informed decisions about your diet and lifestyle.

Cultivating a positive mindset is vital for success. Embrace self-compassion and kindness towards yourself, celebrating every healthy choice and step you take towards your goals. Surround yourself with positivity and inspiration by seeking out success stories of others who have achieved their weight loss goals through dedication and healthy habits.

Visualization can be a powerful tool to stay motivated and focused. Take time each day to visualize yourself at your ideal weight, feeling confident, healthy, and happy. Create a vision board with images that represent your goals, serving as a constant reminder of the rewards that await you on your journey.

Reach out for support and accountability from friends, family, or a weight loss group. Having someone to share your progress and challenges with can provide encouragement and motivation. Consider professional support from a registered dietitian or weight loss coach for personalized guidance.

Celebrate non-scale victories, such as increased energy levels, improved fitness, better sleep, and enhanced overall well-being. Remember that success is not solely measured by the number on the scale.

Learn from setbacks and turn obstacles into opportunities for growth. Analyze the situation, identify triggers, and refine your approach to reinforce your commitment to your goals.

As you progress on your weight loss journey, celebrate achievements and milestones. Establish smaller, attainable goals and treat yourself with rewards upon achieving them. This positive reinforcement will boost your motivation and excitement for continued progress.

Celebrate every step of your transformative journey towards a healthier and happier life. Remember that this is not just about losing weight; it's about embracing a sustainable and positive lifestyle change that will lead to lasting results. Embrace the challenges and victories that come with the "Easy Weight Loss Diet for Maximum Results," and let the journey unfold with determination, patience, and self-belief.

Now that we've discussed the essential components of the roadmap to success on your weight loss journey. It's important to recognize that transforming your lifestyle and achieving your weight loss goals is not a linear process. There will be ups and downs, challenges, and moments of triumph. It's essential to approach your journey with a growth mindset and a willingness to learn from every experience.

As you embark on this transformative path, here are some additional strategies to help you stay on track and maintain a positive mindset:

1. Set Realistic Goals

While it's great to have ambitious long-term goals, it's equally important to set smaller, achievable milestones along the way. Celebrate each milestone as you reach it, and use it as motivation to continue moving forward.

2. Practice Mindful Eating

Mindful eating involves paying full attention to the experience of eating, savoring each bite, and being present in the moment. By eating mindfully, you can better recognize feelings of hunger and fullness, prevent overeating, and enjoy your meals to the fullest.

3. Find Joy in Physical Activity

Exercise doesn't have to be a chore; it can be a source of joy and fun. Explore different types of physical activities and find what you genuinely enjoy. Whether it's dancing, hiking, swimming, or practicing yoga, incorporating activities you love into your routine will make staying active a pleasure, not a burden.

4. Stay Flexible

Life is unpredictable, and there may be occasions when your plans get derailed. Instead of viewing these moments as failures, see them as opportunities to practice flexibility and resilience. Adapt to the situation, and don't be too hard on yourself if things don't go as planned.

5. Reward Yourself with Non-Food Treats

Celebrate your successes with non-food rewards that align with your weight loss goals. Indulge in a soothing massage, treat yourself to a new book, or embark on a day trip to a destination you've always wanted to explore. These non-food treats will reinforce your achievements and provide positive reinforcement for your efforts.

6. Find Supportive Allies

Surround yourself with people who uplift and support you on your weight loss journey. Share your goals with friends and family who will encourage your progress and be there to lend a listening ear when you need it.

7. Reflect and Learn

Regularly take time to reflect on your journey and the progress you've made. Celebrate your successes and identify areas where you can continue to improve. Use past experiences as lessons to inform your future choices and actions.

8. Embrace Change

Transforming your lifestyle involves embracing change and stepping out of your comfort zone. Be open to trying new foods, exploring different exercises, and incorporating healthy habits into your daily routine.

9. Focus on Health, Not Just Weight

While weight loss is a significant goal, remember that your health is the ultimate priority. Focus on the positive impact your dietary and lifestyle changes have on your overall well-being, such as improved energy levels, better sleep, and enhanced mental clarity.

10. Celebrate Every Day

Every day is an opportunity to make progress towards your goals. Celebrate the effort and dedication you put into your journey each day, regardless of the scale's numbers. Recognize that you are taking steps towards a healthier and happier life.

As you implement these strategies and continue following the "Easy Weight Loss Diet for Maximum Results," remember that this is a journey of self-discovery and self-improvement. Celebrate every victory, no matter how small, and keep your focus on the positive changes you are making in your life.

Throughout this chapter, we've explored the roadmap to success, guiding you towards your weight loss goals. By combining determination, patience, and a positive mindset with the principles of the "Easy Weight Loss Diet for Maximum Results," you are equipped with the tools and strategies for a successful and transformative journey. Embrace this opportunity for positive change, and let your dedication lead you to a healthier, happier you.

With every stride you take, remind yourself that this is a path of empowerment and self-improvement. You possess the strength and resilience to reach your weight loss objectives, and with this diet as your compass, you are making significant progress towards a healthier and happier version of yourself. The potential to transform and enhance your life resides within you. Your determination and commitment will propel you to succeed, and as this diet serves as your guiding force, you are well on your way to attain a healthier and happier state.

Let us continue this journey together, step by step, as we explore the delectable and nourishing recipes and practical strategies in the forthcoming chapters. Together, we will turn your weight loss aspirations into a concrete reality. Embrace the opportunities that await, and allow the "Easy Weight Loss Diet for Maximum Results" to empower you to lead the fulfilling life you truly deserve.

Breakfast

Breakfast, often touted as the most important meal of the day, sets the tone for your entire day. It provides the essential fuel and nutrients your body needs to function optimally and kick-starts your metabolism, making it a crucial component of the "Easy Weight Loss Diet for Maximum Results." Let's delve deeper into the key components of a nutritious and satisfying breakfast that will support your weight loss journey and overall well-being.

Breakfast is a time to nourish your body and mind, preparing yourself for the day ahead. By incorporating wholesome and balanced options into your morning meal, you can set yourself up for success and lay the foundation for a healthier lifestyle.

Enjoy a Variety of Fresh Fruits

One of the simplest yet most effective ways to start your day on a healthy note is by enjoying a variety of fresh fruits. From juicy berries and succulent apples to refreshing oranges and tropical delights, the options are endless. Not only do fruits add natural sweetness and vibrant colors to your plate, but they also supply an array of essential vitamins, minerals, and fiber.

Seasonal fruits are a delight for the senses and offer the best taste and nutritional value. They are at their peak freshness, making them the perfect addition to your breakfast. Keep in mind that some fruits, like bananas, become sweeter as they ripen, leading to a higher sugar content. Opt for fruits that are ripe but still firm to maintain a balanced sugar intake.

Choose Sugar-Less or Low-Sugar Cereals

Cereals can be a convenient and tasty breakfast option, but not all cereals are created equal. Many commercial cereals are laden with added sugars, which can lead to energy crashes and increased cravings later in the day. To support your weight loss goals and overall well-being, opt for sugar-less or low-sugar cereal options.

Whole grain or oat-based cereals are excellent choices, providing complex carbohydrates and essential nutrients to fuel your body. Reading nutrition labels can help you make informed decisions about the sugar content in cereals. Moderation is key, and enjoying a bowl of corn flakes or granola in moderation can still fit into your breakfast routine.

Incorporate Low-Fat Dairy Products

Dairy products offer a valuable source of protein and calcium, making them a worthy addition to your breakfast. To maintain a healthy calorie intake, opt for low-fat milk and yogurt. Greek yogurt, in particular, stands out for its high protein content, which can keep you feeling full and satisfied.

Experiment with different ways to include dairy in your breakfast. Enjoy a bowl of yogurt topped with fresh fruits and a sprinkle of nuts for added texture and flavor. Alternatively, add milk to your cereal for a creamy and nutritious start to your day. The protein in dairy products can help stabilize blood sugar levels and curb hunger, making it a wise choice for weight management.

Include Eggs in Your Breakfast

Eggs are a breakfast classic for good reason. These versatile gems are packed with high-quality protein and essential vitamins and minerals. Including eggs in your breakfast can keep you feeling full and energized throughout the morning, making it easier to resist unhealthy snacking before lunch.

Whether you prefer boiled eggs, scrambled eggs, or a light omelet, eggs can be prepared in various delicious ways. To keep the preparation healthier, use a small amount of oil or butter. Add some fresh vegetables to your omelet for an extra nutrient boost.

Opt for Whole Grain Bread

If bread is your breakfast preference, consider opting for whole grain bread over white bread. Whole grain bread retains the nutritious goodness found in the entire grain, including fiber, vitamins, and minerals. The added fiber can support digestive health and promote a feeling of fullness, reducing the likelihood of overeating later in the day.

While enjoying bread in moderation, choose whole grain options to make the most of its nutritional benefits. Spread some natural nut butter or avocado on your toast for a satisfying and wholesome combination.

Embrace Fruit Tea or Green Tea

While coffee and black tea are breakfast favorites for many, consider expanding your horizons with fruit tea or green tea. These herbal teas offer a delightful and healthier alternative. Fruit tea blends come in a variety of flavors, each brimming with antioxidants and natural goodness.

Green tea, renowned for its numerous health benefits, can be a great way to kickstart your day with a dose of antioxidants and a gentle energy boost. By swapping coffee or black tea for these herbal options, you can reduce caffeine intake and support a healthier start to your day.

Add Nuts for Extra Nutrition

Nuts are nutritional powerhouses that can elevate the health profile of your breakfast. Almonds, cashews, walnuts, and more - nuts offer healthy fats, protein, and essential minerals. They can provide sustained energy, making them an excellent addition to your morning meal.

Sprinkle a small handful of nuts on your cereal, mix them into your yogurt, or enjoy them as a standalone snack. Just remember to keep portion sizes in check, as nuts are calorie-dense. The combination of nuts with fruits and dairy in your breakfast will provide a well-rounded and satisfying meal.

In addition to the specific breakfast components, remember that the way you eat is just as important as what you eat. Take the time to savor your breakfast, eat mindfully, and pay attention to your body's hunger and fullness cues. Starting your day with a leisurely and tranquil breakfast establishes a positive ambiance that resonates throughout the rest of your day.

By incorporating these guidelines into your breakfast routine, you can nourish your body, support your weight loss goals, and set yourself up for success throughout the day. Breakfast truly is the foundation for a healthier, happier you in the "Easy Weight Loss Diet for Maximum Results."

Enjoy this opportunity to start each day on a positive and nutritious note, and let your breakfast be a delicious stepping stone toward achieving your wellness aspirations.

Lunch

Lunch is a vital meal that provides a midday refueling and sustains your energy levels for the remainder of the day. As a key part of the "Easy Weight Loss Diet for Maximum Results," lunch should be a well-balanced and satisfying combination of various food groups. In this chapter, we will explore the recommended components of a healthy lunch that will support your weight loss journey and keep you feeling nourished and energized.

A well-structured lunch is essential for maintaining steady energy levels and preventing unhealthy snacking later in the day. By focusing on nutrient-dense and satisfying foods, you can avoid post-lunch slumps and maintain productivity and focus throughout the afternoon.

The Foundation: A Balanced Meal

A nutritious lunch should encompass a mix of proteins, vegetables, legumes, fruits, and healthy beverages. Strive to create a plate that represents a rainbow of colors and a variety of textures. The goal is to achieve a well-rounded meal that offers a diverse range of nutrients to fuel your body.

Proteins for Sustained Energy

Proteins play a crucial role in maintaining energy levels and supporting weight loss. They keep you feeling fuller for longer, reducing the likelihood of overeating throughout the afternoon. Including a source of lean protein in your lunch can help you feel satisfied and curb unnecessary snacking.

Consider incorporating grilled chicken, turkey, or fish as a protein-rich option. If you follow a plant-based diet, explore dishes like chickpea salad, lentil stew, or tofu stir-fry.

These plant-based protein sources not only contribute to your protein intake but also provide essential vitamins and minerals.

Embrace the Power of Vegetables

Vegetables are a nutritional powerhouse and an essential component of any healthy lunch. They are rich in vitamins, minerals, and fiber, promoting digestive health and overall well-being. Including a variety of colorful vegetables in your lunch not only enhances the visual appeal of your plate but also maximizes the nutritional value of your meal.

Create a refreshing salad by combining mixed greens, bell peppers, cherry tomatoes, cucumber, and grated carrots. Alternatively, opt for cooked vegetables like steamed broccoli, roasted sweet potatoes, or stir-fried mixed vegetables. Experiment with different seasonings and dressings to add exciting flavors to your vegetables.

Lentils and Legumes for Plant-Based Protein

Lentils and legumes are not only rich in protein but also high in fiber, making them a satisfying addition to your lunch. They help stabilize blood sugar levels and support healthy digestion, which can prevent energy crashes and hunger pangs later in the day.

Lentil soups, bean salads, and hummus wraps are some delicious and filling ways to incorporate legumes into your lunch. Experiment with different herbs and spices to enhance the flavors of these plant-based protein sources.

Fruits for Natural Sweetness

Fresh fruits provide a naturally sweet and refreshing touch to your lunch. They are packed with vitamins, minerals, and antioxidants, offering a nourishing boost to your day. Including a serving of seasonal fruits in your lunch not only adds natural sweetness but also contributes to your daily fruit intake.

Slice up some fresh fruits like apples, berries, or oranges as a delightful side to your lunch. You can also enjoy a fruit salad with a mix of your favorite fruits for a more diverse and colorful option.

Stay Hydrated with Water and Pure Fruit Juice

Aim to drink water throughout the day, and especially during lunch, to keep your body well-hydrated. Staying hydrated can also help control hunger and prevent overeating.

While water should be your primary beverage, you can also include 100% pure fruit juice as an occasional treat. However, be cautious of fruit drinks that contain added sugars, as they can contribute to empty calories and hinder your weight loss efforts.

Choose Low-Fat Dairy Products

If you enjoy dairy products, opt for low-fat or reduced-fat options. Low-fat yogurt, cottage cheese, or a small serving of cheese can be included in your lunch to add a creamy and satisfying element. These dairy products provide calcium and protein while being mindful of calorie intake.

Greek yogurt with a drizzle of honey and fresh berries can make a delightful and nutritious addition to your lunch. Alternatively, a small serving of low-fat cheese paired with whole-grain crackers can be a satisfying midday snack.

Rice: Moderation and Healthy Choices

Rice can be part of a healthy lunch, but it's essential to exercise moderation and choose healthier varieties. Brown rice, known for its higher fiber content and more substantial nutritional profile, is a better option compared to white rice.

If you prefer white rice, try to keep the portion size in check to avoid excessive carbohydrate intake. Incorporate other whole grains like quinoa, barley, or bulgur for added variety and nutrients.

Listening to Your Appetite

A key principle of the "Easy Weight Loss Diet for Maximum Results" is to pay attention to your body's hunger and fullness cues. Listen to your appetite during lunch and eat until you feel comfortably satisfied, rather than overly full.

By eating mindfully and being in tune with your body's signals, you can prevent overeating and ensure that you are nourishing yourself adequately.

Explore Food Options in Detail

In the upcoming chapters, we will delve into greater detail about the specific foods you can include in your diet to support your weight loss goals. We will cover a wide range of foods that can be incorporated into different meals throughout the day. From nutrient-rich breakfast ideas to satisfying lunch options, delectable dinner choices, and delightful snacks, you will find a diverse array of foods that align with the "Easy Weight Loss Diet for Maximum Results."

Embrace the opportunity to create balanced and delicious meals that fuel your body and support your weight loss journey. By incorporating a variety of nutrients and flavors, you can make each meal a delightful and nourishing experience every day.

Dinner

In the "Easy Weight Loss Diet for Maximum Results," the emphasis is on giving your digestive system a well-deserved rest during the evening hours. Dinner is a crucial meal of the day, but the approach to it differs from breakfast and lunch. Instead of indulging in heavy or large meals, this diet encourages you to opt for something light and easily digestible in the evening. In this chapter, we will explore the reasons behind this approach and the benefits it offers in your weight loss journey and overall health.

The Importance of Light Evening Meals

Dinner time is when many people tend to overeat or consume heavy and calorie-laden foods, which can lead to weight gain and digestive discomfort. Eating large quantities of food right before bedtime does not give your body sufficient time to process and metabolize the nutrients properly. This can disrupt your sleep and affect the body's ability to burn calories efficiently.

By opting for a light dinner, you allow your digestive system to work more effectively, promoting better digestion and absorption of nutrients. Additionally, this approach can prevent you from feeling sluggish or bloated in the evening, allowing you to enjoy a restful night's sleep.

The Main Focus on Breakfast and Lunch

In the "Easy Weight Loss Diet for Maximum Results," the primary focus is on breakfast and lunch. These meals are considered the foundation of your daily nutrition and energy needs. Breakfast sets the tone for your day, providing you with the necessary nutrients and energy to kickstart your morning. Lunch sustains you through the rest of the day, keeping you fueled and focused on your tasks.

Both breakfast and lunch allow you to eat as much as you like from the foods that are allowed in this diet. This flexibility ensures that you feel satisfied and nourished during the most active part of your day.

The Importance of Portion Control

While breakfast and lunch encourage a sense of abundance and satisfaction, dinner takes a different approach by focusing on portion control. By consuming a lighter evening meal, you can better manage your calorie intake and avoid the excess calories that can lead to weight gain.

Portion control is essential in maintaining a balanced diet and ensuring that you are eating within your body's caloric needs. It helps you strike the right balance between nourishing your body and preventing overeating.

Choosing the Right Foods for Dinner

In the evening, it's best to select foods that are easy to digest and gentle on your stomach. Opt for foods that are nutrient-dense and provide essential vitamins and minerals without being heavy or calorie-dense.

Salads are an excellent option for a light and refreshing dinner. Load up on fresh vegetables, leafy greens, and a source of lean protein. You can add some nuts or seeds for an extra crunch and a boost of healthy fats.

Fruits are another suitable choice for a light evening meal. Opt for fruits with low sugar content, such as apples, berries, and citrus fruits. They provide natural sweetness and are packed with vitamins and antioxidants.

Low-fat dairy products like low-fat milk or low-fat yogurt can also be included in your dinner. They are a good source of protein and calcium, contributing to your overall nutritional needs.

Nuts can make a satisfying and nutritious evening snack. They offer healthy fats and protein, helping you feel satiated without overloading your digestive system.

The Benefits of a Light Evening Meal

Choosing a light dinner has numerous benefits for your weight loss journey and overall well-being. By consuming fewer calories in the evening, you create a calorie deficit that can aid in weight loss. Additionally, eating lighter meals in the evening can improve digestion and prevent discomfort like indigestion and heartburn. Moreover, a light dinner can lead to better sleep quality. When your digestive system isn't working overtime to process heavy foods, you are more likely to experience restful and undisturbed sleep.

The Role of Mindful Eating

Mindful eating is an essential aspect of this diet, even during dinner time. It involves paying attention to your body's hunger and fullness cues, as well as savoring and enjoying each bite.

By eating mindfully, you can prevent overeating and make conscious choices about the foods you consume.

Listen to your body and eat until you feel comfortably satisfied, rather than overly full. Eating slowly and mindfully allows your body to signal when it has had enough, reducing the likelihood of overindulging.

A Balanced and Sustainable Approach

The "Easy Weight Loss Diet for Maximum Results" emphasizes a balanced and sustainable approach to eating. By focusing on light dinners, you give your body the opportunity to rest and recover in the evening, setting the stage for a healthier lifestyle. While dinner may be lighter, breakfast and lunch provide ample opportunities to enjoy a variety of foods that nourish your body and support your weight loss goals. By following this balanced approach, you can create a harmonious relationship with food and promote long-term success in your weight loss journey.

In the upcoming chapters, we will delve further into the specifics of the recommended foods for breakfast, lunch, and dinner. You will find a diverse range of options that cater to your taste preferences and dietary needs, all while supporting your weight loss efforts.

Vegetables

In the "Easy Weight Loss Diet for Maximum Results," vegetables take center stage as essential components of your daily meals. These nutrient-packed wonders are not only delicious and versatile but also play a vital role in your weight loss journey. In this chapter, we will explore the various qualities of vegetables, their impressive nutritional value, their ease of digestion, and the multitude of benefits they offer in promoting weight loss and overall health.

The Nutritional Value of Vegetables

Vegetables are nutritional powerhouses, providing a wide array of essential vitamins, minerals, and other nutrients that are crucial for your body's optimal functioning. They are rich in fiber, antioxidants, and phytochemicals, which contribute to their numerous health benefits.

Fiber: One of the key features of vegetables is their high fiber content. Dietary fiber aids in digestion, promotes a feeling of fullness, and helps regulate blood sugar levels. By keeping you satiated, fiber reduces the likelihood of overeating and supports your weight loss efforts.

Vitamins and Minerals: Vegetables are abundant sources of vitamins like vitamin A, C, K, and various B vitamins. They also contain essential minerals such as potassium, magnesium, and calcium, which are vital for maintaining overall health.

Antioxidants: Antioxidants found in vegetables help neutralize harmful free radicals in the body, which can cause cellular damage. By reducing oxidative stress, antioxidants support cellular health and may have a positive impact on weight management.

Phytochemicals: These naturally occurring compounds in vegetables have been linked to various health benefits, including reducing inflammation and supporting cardiovascular health.

The Digestive Friendliness of Vegetables

Vegetables are inherently easy to digest, making them a fantastic addition to your weight loss diet. Their fiber content aids in promoting regular bowel movements and supporting a healthy gut. By supporting proper digestion and bowel health, vegetables prevent digestive discomfort and bloating, which can be obstacles in your weight loss journey.

Vegetables and Weight Loss

Vegetables are hailed as an essential tool for weight loss for several reasons:

1. Low in Calories: Most vegetables are low in calories, allowing you to consume larger portions without consuming excessive calories. This means you can feel satisfied and full while staying within your caloric limits.

2. High in Fiber: As mentioned earlier, vegetables' high fiber content promotes satiety and prevents overeating, making them a great ally in your efforts to shed pounds.

3. Nutrient Density: Despite being low in calories, vegetables are incredibly nutrient-dense. They provide your body with essential nutrients, ensuring that you get the necessary vitamins and minerals while managing your weight.

4. Water Content: Many vegetables have a high water content, contributing to their low calorie and high volume nature. This water content adds to their satiety factor and keeps you hydrated.

5. Slow Digestion: The fiber and complex carbohydrates in vegetables lead to slower digestion, helping maintain stable blood sugar levels and preventing sudden spikes in hunger.

Variety in Vegetables

One of the greatest advantages of incorporating vegetables into your diet is the vast array of options available. From leafy greens like spinach, kale, and lettuce to colorful bell peppers, carrots, and tomatoes, the choices are endless. This variety ensures that you can enjoy different flavors and textures, preventing meal monotony and making your weight loss journey more enjoyable.

How to Incorporate More Vegetables into Your Diet

To reap the full benefits of vegetables, aim to include them in every meal. Here are some practical tips to increase your vegetable intake:

1. Start Your Day with Veggies: Add vegetables to your breakfast by including them in omelets, smoothies, or as a side dish.

2. Create Colorful Salads: Make salads with a variety of vegetables, leafy greens, and a source of lean protein. Dress them with a light vinaigrette for a refreshing and satisfying meal.

3. Veggie-Loaded Lunches: Prepare vegetable-packed wraps, sandwiches, or grain bowls for your midday meal. Include a mix of raw and cooked vegetables for a delightful texture.

4. Snack on Veggies: Keep cut-up vegetables like carrots, cucumbers, and celery sticks on hand for quick and healthy snacks.

5. Get Creative with Dinners: Experiment with vegetable-based pasta alternatives like zucchini noodles, or make cauliflower rice for a low-carb option.

6. Grill or Roast Vegetables: Grilling or roasting vegetables brings out their natural flavors and adds depth to your meals.

7. Veggie Soups and Stews: Prepare hearty soups and stews with an abundance of vegetables for a warm and comforting meal.

Mindful Cooking and Preparing

When cooking vegetables, opt for methods that preserve their nutritional value. Lightly steam, sauté, or roast them to retain their nutrients and natural flavors. Avoid deep frying or overcooking, as these methods can diminish the nutritional content of vegetables.

The Benefits of Vegetable-Rich Diet

Incorporating vegetables into your diet offers a myriad of benefits:

1. Weight Management: The low-calorie and high-fiber nature of vegetables contribute to weight loss and weight management. They help you feel full and satisfied without consuming excessive calories.

2. Improved Digestion: Vegetables' fiber content aids digestion and promotes a healthy gut, preventing digestive discomfort.

3. Enhanced Nutrient Intake: Vegetables are abundant sources of essential vitamins, minerals, and antioxidants, contributing to overall health and wellness.

4. Heart Health: The nutrients in vegetables are linked to improved heart health, reducing the risk of cardiovascular diseases.

5. Blood Sugar Control: The fiber and complex carbohydrates in vegetables help stabilize blood sugar levels, making them beneficial for individuals with diabetes.

6. Reduced Inflammation: The antioxidants and phytochemicals in vegetables have anti-inflammatory properties, benefiting overall health.

Vegetables offer an array of nutrients, support healthy digestion, and play a significant role in weight management. By incorporating a colorful and diverse selection of vegetables into your meals, you can enjoy a satisfying and nourishing diet that fosters weight loss and boosts overall well-being.

In the next chapters, we will continue to explore the benefits of other food groups and how they complement your weight loss journey. Remember, a balanced and mindful approach to eating, with an abundance of vegetables, will pave the way to your desired health and wellness goals.

Fruits

In the "Easy Weight Loss Diet for Maximum Results," fruits hold a special place as vibrant and wholesome additions to your daily meals. These naturally sweet delights not only satisfy your taste buds but also offer a plethora of health benefits. In this chapter, we will delve into the extensive benefits of fruits, explore their rich nutritional value, vitamins, and various qualities that make them indispensable allies in your weight loss journey.

The Bountiful Benefits of Fruits

Fruits are a gift from nature, packed with goodness and nourishment. They provide a wide range of health benefits, contributing to overall well-being and vitality:

1. Rich in Vitamins: Fruits are abundant sources of essential vitamins, including vitamin C, vitamin A, vitamin K, and various B vitamins. These vitamins play crucial roles in immune function, vision, skin health, and metabolic processes.

2. Loaded with Minerals: Fruits contain important minerals like potassium, magnesium, and calcium, which are vital for maintaining heart health, nerve function, and bone strength.

3. Antioxidant Powerhouse: Fruits are rich in antioxidants, such as flavonoids and polyphenols, which combat oxidative stress and protect your cells from damage caused by free radicals.

4. Hydration and Fiber: Many fruits have a high water content, contributing to hydration. Additionally, fruits are an excellent source of dietary fiber, promoting digestive health and supporting weight management.

5. Natural Energy: The natural sugars in fruits provide a quick and sustainable source of energy, making them a fantastic choice for a midday pick-me-up.

The Nutritional Value of Fruits

Fruits offer an impressive array of essential nutrients that contribute to overall health:

1. Vitamin C: Found abundantly in citrus fruits like oranges, lemons, and grapefruits, vitamin C supports immune function, collagen production, and acts as a powerful antioxidant, protecting the body from harmful free radicals.

2. Vitamin A: Fruits like mangoes, papayas, and apricots are rich sources of vitamin A, which is essential for maintaining healthy vision, supporting the immune system, and promoting skin health.

3. Potassium: Bananas, oranges, and avocados are excellent sources of potassium, a vital mineral that plays a crucial role in regulating blood pressure, heart health, and muscle function.

4. Fiber: Apples, pears, and berries are packed with dietary fiber, which aids in digestion, promotes satiety, and helps regulate blood sugar levels, all contributing factors to weight management.

5. Antioxidants: Berries, such as blueberries, strawberries, and raspberries, are renowned for their antioxidant content, which helps combat oxidative stress and reduces the risk of chronic diseases.

Fruits and Weight Loss

Incorporating a variety of fruits into your weight loss diet can be highly beneficial:

1. Low in Calories: Most fruits are naturally low in calories, making them an ideal choice for those looking to manage their caloric intake while feeling satisfied and nourished.

2. Satiety: The fiber content in fruits promotes a feeling of fullness and satiety, reducing the likelihood of overeating and aiding in weight management efforts.

3. Natural Sweetness: Fruits provide a delicious and nutritious alternative to processed sugars and sugary snacks, making them a guilt-free option for satisfying your sweet cravings.

4. Hydration: Many fruits have high water content, contributing to hydration and ensuring your body stays refreshed and energized throughout the day.

5. Nutrient Density: Despite their low caloric content, fruits are nutrient-dense, meaning they are rich in essential vitamins, minerals, and antioxidants that support overall health and well-being.

Citrus Fruits and Their Impact on Weight Loss

Citrus fruits, including oranges, lemons, grapefruits, and tangerines, hold a special place in the realm of weight loss. These zesty fruits offer a unique combination of nutrients and compounds that can aid in shedding unwanted pounds:

1. Vitamin C: Citrus fruits are particularly rich in vitamin C, an essential nutrient that supports the immune system and helps the body absorb iron, crucial for energy production and metabolism.

2. Hydration: With their high water content, citrus fruits contribute to hydration, making them an excellent choice for a refreshing snack during hot weather or after physical activity.

3. Low in Calories: Citrus fruits are relatively low in calories, making them a smart option for those aiming to manage their weight while still enjoying flavorful and satisfying snacks.

4. Natural Detoxification: Citrus fruits contain natural compounds that support the body's detoxification processes, helping to flush out toxins and waste, which can contribute to better digestion and weight management.

5. Blood Sugar Regulation: Citrus fruits have a low glycemic index, meaning they have a minimal impact on blood sugar levels. This can be beneficial for individuals looking to stabilize their blood sugar and avoid spikes that can lead to cravings and overeating.

Incorporating Fruits into Your Diet

To make the most of the benefits that fruits offer, aim to include a variety of fruits in your daily meals:

1. Snack on Fruits: Keep a bowl of fresh fruits on your kitchen counter or desk for easy and healthy snacking throughout the day.

2. Fruit Smoothies: Blend your favorite fruits with low-fat yogurt or plant-based milk for a refreshing and nutrient-packed smoothie.

3. Fruits in Salads: Add sliced apples, berries, or citrus segments to your salads for a burst of flavor and color.

4. Fruit Parfaits: Layer fruits with Greek yogurt and granola for a delightful and nutritious dessert option.

5. Fresh Fruit Desserts: Enjoy fresh fruit salads or grilled fruit for a naturally sweet and wholesome dessert.

Fruits are nature's bountiful gift to us, brimming with essential nutrients, antioxidants, and natural sweetness. By incorporating a colorful assortment of fruits into your diet, you can enjoy a host of health benefits while supporting your weight loss journey. Whether as a standalone snack or as a delectable addition to your meals, fruits bring both nourishment and delight to your table. Embrace the vibrancy and richness of fruits as you continue your path to a healthier, happier you. With an array of fruits at your fingertips, you have the power to make your weight loss journey a flavorful and rewarding experience.

Healthy Meat

Incorporating healthy meat into your diet can be a valuable strategy for achieving weight loss and maintaining overall well-being. When consumed in moderation and prepared in a healthy manner, various types of meat can offer an array of essential nutrients that contribute to a balanced diet. This chapter will delve into the benefits and significance of different types of healthy meat, including grass-fed beef, organic chicken, goat meat, grass-fed lamb, rabbit meat, game meat and turkey meat.

1. Grass-Fed Beef

One of the primary healthy meat choices is grass-fed beef, which is sourced from cattle that graze on natural grass rather than being raised on grain-based diets. Grass-fed beef is an excellent source of essential nutrients, including protein, iron, zinc, and various B vitamins. The fat in grass-fed beef tends to be healthier than conventional grain-fed beef, with a more favorable ratio of omega-3 to omega-6 fatty acids. Additionally, the removal of excess fat from the meat further promotes its health benefits.

The meat from animals no older than two years is preferred because it typically contains more tender and lean cuts. Consuming grass-fed beef can aid in maintaining muscle mass during weight loss, making it a valuable addition to a balanced diet.

Not only does grass-fed beef offer numerous health advantages, but it also has positive environmental impacts. Grass-fed farming practices promote more sustainable and ethical approaches to meat production, as they contribute to lower greenhouse gas emissions and less soil degradation compared to conventional feedlot operations.

2. Organic Chicken

Organic chicken, particularly chicken breast, is another wholesome option for individuals looking to lose weight and enhance their health. Organic chicken is raised without the use of antibiotics or growth hormones, ensuring a cleaner and healthier meat source. Chicken breast, in particular, is low in fat and high in protein, making it an ideal choice for those aiming to shed pounds.

Protein from organic chicken supports muscle maintenance and repair, boosts metabolism, and keeps you feeling full for longer periods, reducing the chances of overeating. It also contains essential amino acids that aid in various bodily functions, including immune support and tissue repair.

Incorporating organic chicken into your diet can also have positive effects on the environment. Supporting organic farming practices encourages sustainable agriculture, reduces the use of harmful chemicals, and promotes the ethical treatment of animals.

3. Goat Meat

Goat meat, often referred to as "chevon" or "mutton," is a lesser-known but highly nutritious type of healthy meat. It is a common staple in many cultures and is gradually gaining popularity worldwide due to its unique flavor and impressive nutritional profile. Goat meat is a rich source of high-quality protein, iron, and vitamin B12.

Compared to beef and lamb, goat meat is leaner and contains less saturated fat, which can be beneficial for those watching their fat intake while trying to lose weight. Furthermore, goat meat is rich in conjugated linoleic acid (CLA), a type of healthy fat known for its potential health benefits, including weight loss and reduced inflammation.

In addition to its nutritional benefits, goat meat also has ecological advantages. Goats are generally hardy animals that can thrive in harsh environments, and their grazing habits can help manage vegetation, reducing the risk of wildfires and promoting biodiversity.

4. grass-fed lamb

Similar to grass-fed beef, lamb raised on a natural grass diet offers numerous health advantages. Although lamb should be eaten in moderation due to its relatively higher fat content compared to other lean meats, it can still be part of a healthy diet. Grass-fed lamb is a good source of protein, iron, zinc, and vitamin B12.

The key to incorporating grass-fed lamb into a weight loss plan is to be mindful of portion sizes and to balance it with plenty of vegetables and other nutrient-dense foods. The protein and nutrients found in lamb contribute to muscle maintenance and overall health, but excessive consumption may hinder weight loss efforts.

5. Rabbit Meat

Rabbit meat, often referred to as "coney" or "lapin," is a lean and tender meat option that can be a valuable addition to a weight loss diet. Rabbit meat is an excellent source of high-quality protein while being low in calories and fat. It is also rich in essential nutrients like vitamin B12, selenium, and phosphorus.

Incorporating rabbit meat into your meals can help you stay satiated with fewer calories, making it easier to control your overall calorie intake and support weight loss. Additionally, the nutrients in rabbit meat promote energy production, cell repair, and immune function, all of which are essential during a weight loss journey.

6. Game Meat

Game meats, including venison, elk, bison, and wild boar, provide an assortment of benefits similar to those found in grass-fed meats. These animals typically roam freely and eat natural diets, resulting in leaner and healthier meat choices. Game meats are excellent sources of protein, iron, and zinc, and they often contain lower levels of fat compared to conventionally raised meats.

Incorporating game meat into your diet can add variety and new flavors while providing essential nutrients to support your weight loss goals. The increased protein content aids in maintaining muscle mass during weight loss, while the lower fat content contributes to a healthier overall diet.

Notably, game meats can contribute to conservation efforts by supporting sustainable hunting practices and wildlife management. When managed responsibly, hunting can help control animal populations and maintain ecological balance in certain regions.

7. Turkey Meat

Turkey meat offers a plethora of health benefits, making it an excellent choice for those aiming for weight loss and overall well-being. This lean and protein-rich meat is low in fat and calories, making it a satisfying option for weight-conscious individuals. The high protein content in turkey meat helps promote satiety, reducing the likelihood of overeating and aiding in weight management.

Additionally, turkey meat is a great source of essential nutrients, including vitamins B6 and B12, which play a vital role in metabolism and energy production. Moreover, it contains selenium, a powerful antioxidant that supports a healthy immune system and protects cells from oxidative stress. Incorporating turkey meat into a balanced diet can provide the necessary nutrients while supporting weight loss goals, making it a delectable and nutritious addition to any healthy eating plan.

Healthy meat, when consumed as part of a balanced diet and prepared in a healthy manner, can be a valuable component of a weight loss plan. Grass-fed beef, organic chicken, goat meat, grass-fed lamb, rabbit meat, and game meat each offer unique nutritional benefits that contribute to overall health and well-being. By being mindful of portion sizes and pairing these meats with a variety of nutrient-dense foods, you can create a diet that supports weight loss while enjoying the savory flavors and health benefits these meats have to offer.

With informed choices and a focus on sustainability, incorporating healthy meat into your diet can not only benefit your health but also contribute to a healthier planet for future generations.

Seafood

Seafood is not only a powerhouse of nutrition but also a delightful addition to any meal. Its delectable flavors and versatility in cooking methods make it a favorite among food enthusiasts. Let's delve into the exceptional qualities of various types of seafood, with a main focus on white-fleshed fish, including salmon, cod, flounder, Alaskan Pollock, shrimp, crab and carp.

Salmon

Salmon's reputation as a delicious and healthy fish is well-deserved. Its tender flesh and distinct flavor make it a popular choice for seafood lovers. Moreover, salmon is incredibly versatile and can be prepared in various ways - from grilling and baking to pan-searing and poaching. The culinary appeal of salmon extends to various cuisines worldwide. In Asian cuisine, it is often marinated with flavorful sauces and spices, while in Western dishes, it is commonly paired with fresh herbs and citrus flavors. Additionally, smoked salmon adds a distinctive touch to salads, pasta dishes, and even breakfast spreads.

Cod

With its mild taste and delicate texture, cod is a crowd-pleaser, particularly for those who are new to seafood. Its versatility shines through in the kitchen, making it an excellent choice for quick and easy meals. Cod can be baked with a drizzle of olive oil and herbs, pan-fried with a light coating of breadcrumbs, or even steamed to preserve its natural moisture. In Mediterranean cuisines, cod is often featured in hearty stews and casseroles, incorporating an array of vegetables and aromatic spices. This versatility allows home cooks to experiment with different flavors and cooking methods to suit their taste preferences.

Flounder

Flounder's tender, flaky texture and subtle taste have earned it a spot on the menus of gourmet restaurants and home kitchens alike. Its delicate nature makes it perfect for a variety of cooking styles. Flounder can be sautéed with garlic and butter, roasted with a medley of vegetables, or simply grilled with a squeeze of lemon for a refreshing and healthy meal. In coastal cuisines, flounder is often celebrated in traditional recipes, where it is stuffed with fresh herbs and seasoned breadcrumbs before being baked to perfection. Its ability to absorb flavors makes it an ideal canvas for culinary creativity.

Alaskan Pollock

Alaskan Pollock is a highly versatile white-fleshed fish that is commonly sold in grocery stores and seafood markets. It is a mild-tasting fish with a firm texture, making it suitable for a wide range of recipes. Alaskan Pollock is often used to make fish sticks, fish filets, and imitation crab meat. It can be grilled, baked, fried, or poached, making it a convenient and delicious addition to any meal. This sustainable seafood choice is not only flavorful but also highly nutritious. Alaskan Pollock is a good source of protein, vitamins, and minerals, including omega-3 fatty acids, which are beneficial for heart health and brain function. Its low-calorie and low-fat content make it a great option for those seeking weight loss and maintaining a healthy diet.

Shrimp

Shrimp's succulent taste and delightful bite make it a culinary delight across the globe. Whether sautéed, grilled, or boiled, shrimp is a versatile ingredient that adds an elegant touch to any dish. In a matter of minutes, shrimp can be transformed into an exquisite appetizer, a mouthwatering main course, or a delightful addition to pasta dishes and salads. In Southeast Asian cuisines, shrimp takes center stage in vibrant curries, stir-fries, and noodle dishes, infused with aromatic spices and coconut milk. In the Americas, shrimp is often celebrated in classic dishes such as shrimp scampi, jambalaya, and ceviche.

Crab

Crab's sweet and delicate flavor is a true seafood indulgence. Whether enjoyed as succulent crab legs or lump crabmeat, this crustacean offers a unique taste experience. Crab can be steamed, boiled, or pan-seared to showcase its natural sweetness and tenderness. In coastal regions, crab is a staple in seafood boils and feasts, served with corn on the cob, potatoes, and various seasonings. Crab cakes, a beloved dish in many cuisines, are a harmonious blend of crabmeat, breadcrumbs, and spices, showcasing the delectable taste of this crustacean.

Carp

Carp fish can indeed be a beneficial addition to a weight loss diet. This freshwater fish is not only delectable but also offers various health advantages. Carp is a low-calorie and low-fat fish, making it a suitable choice for individuals looking to shed excess pounds. Packed with high-quality protein, carp helps promote feelings of fullness and satiety, which can prevent overeating and support weight management efforts. Additionally, it is rich in essential nutrients such as omega-3 fatty acids, which have been linked to improved heart health and reduced inflammation. Omega-3s also play a role in enhancing metabolism and fat burning, further aiding in weight loss. With its delicious taste and numerous health benefits, incorporating carp fish into your diet can be a smart and flavorful way to support your weight loss journey.

Seafood's tantalizing flavors, coupled with its abundance of health benefits, make it an essential part of any wholesome diet. White-fleshed fish such as salmon, cod, flounder, Alaskan Pollock, shrimp, and crab offer not only a culinary delight but also contribute to weight loss and overall well-being. The ease and quickness with which seafood can be cooked add to its appeal for busy individuals and home cooks alike. With a myriad of cooking methods and flavor profiles to choose from, seafood provides endless possibilities in the kitchen. From exotic spices and herbs to simple lemon and butter, each preparation brings out the best in these succulent offerings from the sea.

It comes as no surprise that many healthy cuisines around the world emphasize the use of seafood. From the Mediterranean's heart-healthy seafood-rich diet to Japan's traditional sushi and sashimi, seafood is celebrated for its role in promoting longevity and vitality. When incorporating seafood into your diet, always opt for sustainably sourced options to support healthy fisheries and protect marine ecosystems.

Legumes

Legumes, the diverse family of plants that includes beans, lentils, chickpeas, peas, and more, have been a staple in diets across the globe for centuries. These humble legumes offer a plethora of health benefits and play a vital role in promoting weight loss. In this chapter, we will explore the exceptional qualities of various legumes, their nutritional value, and how they can aid in shedding those extra pounds.

Nutritional Powerhouses

Legumes are nutritional powerhouses, rich in essential nutrients that contribute to overall well-being. They are an excellent source of plant-based protein, making them a valuable option for vegetarians and vegans seeking to meet their protein needs. Unlike animal-based protein sources, legumes are naturally low in fat and cholesterol, making them heart-healthy choices.

One of the remarkable aspects of legumes is their high fiber content. Fiber not only aids digestion but also provides a feeling of fullness, reducing overall calorie intake. This satiety effect is essential for weight loss, as it helps control hunger and prevents overeating. Additionally, the soluble fiber in legumes helps lower LDL cholesterol levels, reducing the risk of heart disease.

Promoting Weight Loss

Legumes are incredibly beneficial for individuals striving to achieve weight loss goals. As mentioned earlier, their fiber content helps create a sense of fullness and satiety. When included in meals, legumes can lead to reduced appetite and better portion control, making it easier to adhere to a calorie deficit for weight loss.

Moreover, legumes have a low glycemic index, meaning they cause a slow and steady rise in blood sugar levels. This slow digestion of the complex carbohydrates found in legumes helps stabilize blood sugar, preventing sudden spikes and crashes that can lead to unhealthy food cravings.

Beyond their fiber and slow-digesting carbs, legumes are an excellent source of high-quality protein. Protein plays a crucial role in maintaining lean muscle mass while promoting fat loss. Additionally, legumes contain essential amino acids that support various bodily functions, including muscle repair and hormone production.

Various Legumes and Their Benefits:

1. Black Beans

Black beans, with their dark color and earthy taste, are a popular legume in Latin American cuisine. They are an excellent source of protein, fiber, and essential minerals like iron and magnesium. Consuming black beans can enhance heart health, regulate blood sugar levels, and support weight management by promoting a feeling of fullness.

2. Lentils

Lentils come in various colors, including green, red, and brown, and boast a rich nutritional profile. They are a fantastic source of protein, iron, and folate. The soluble fiber in lentils helps in lowering cholesterol levels and controlling blood sugar, making them an ideal addition to a weight loss diet.

3. Chickpeas (Garbanzo Beans)

Chickpeas are a versatile legume used in various cuisines worldwide. Chickpeas aid in weight loss by promoting fullness and reducing the risk of overeating. Moreover, they contain resistant starch, a type of carbohydrate that resists digestion, leading to increased fat oxidation and improved weight management.

4. Peas

Peas, whether green or yellow, are a delightful and nutritious addition to any meal. They are rich in fiber, vitamin C, and vitamin K. The fiber content in peas supports digestive health and helps regulate blood sugar levels, contributing to weight management. Peas also contain antioxidants that protect the body from free radicals and inflammation.

5. Kidney Beans

Kidney beans, with their distinct shape and color, are an excellent source of plant-based protein, fiber, and iron. They can help stabilize blood sugar levels and prevent cravings, aiding in weight loss efforts. Additionally, kidney beans are rich in resistant starch, making them a valuable ally in weight management.

6. Navy Beans

Navy beans, also known as haricot beans, are small, white beans that pack a nutritional punch. They are high in fiber, protein, and essential minerals like potassium and magnesium. Navy beans can help curb appetite and maintain steady energy levels, making them beneficial for weight loss. Furthermore, their high magnesium content supports muscle function and helps regulate blood pressure.

7. Adzuki Beans

Adzuki beans, commonly used in Asian desserts and dishes, are a rich source of protein, fiber, and iron. These beans can assist in weight management by supporting a feeling of fullness and providing sustained energy. Adzuki beans are also known to support kidney health and promote detoxification in the body.

8. Mung Beans

Mung beans are a popular ingredient in Asian cuisine, often used in salads and stir-fries. They are low in calories and high in fiber and protein, making them an excellent choice for weight loss. Mung beans also contain antioxidants that contribute to overall health and protect the body from oxidative stress.

9. Pinto Beans

Pinto beans are an excellent source of protein, fiber, and various essential minerals, including manganese, which supports metabolism and bone health. Pinto beans' ability to stabilize blood sugar levels can help regulate appetite and prevent sudden hunger pangs.

10. Cowpeas (Black-eyed Peas)

Cowpeas, commonly known as black-eyed peas, are rich in protein, fiber, and folate. They are low in calories and fat, making them a weight-friendly option. Black-eyed peas can aid in weight management by promoting fullness and providing sustained energy. Additionally, they contain phytonutrients with antioxidant properties.

Incorporating Legumes into Your Diet

The versatility of legumes makes them easy to incorporate into a variety of dishes. They can be used in soups, stews, salads, curries, and even baked goods. Replace meat with legumes in traditional recipes or create new dishes centered around these nutrient-packed gems.

A Word of Caution

While legumes offer numerous health benefits, some individuals may experience digestive discomfort, such as gas and bloating, when consuming them. It's essential to introduce legumes gradually into your diet and drink plenty of water to aid digestion. Additionally, individuals with specific dietary restrictions or medical conditions should consult with a healthcare professional or a registered dietitian before making significant changes to their diet.

Legumes are a gift from nature, providing an abundance of nutrients and aiding in weight loss efforts. From protein-packed black beans to fiber-rich lentils and chickpeas, each legume brings its unique nutritional benefits to the table. Including a variety of legumes in your diet can lead to better overall health and support your weight loss journey.

Enjoy the delicious flavors and nourishing qualities of legumes, and embrace the benefits they bring to your body and well-being. Whether you're a seasoned legume enthusiast or new to exploring their goodness, there's a legume for everyone to savor and enjoy on the path to a healthier

lifestyle.

Nuts

Nuts are not only a delicious and convenient snack but also a powerhouse of nutrients that can support your weight loss journey. These tiny yet mighty treats are rich in healthy fats, protein, fiber, vitamins, and minerals, making them an essential component of a balanced diet. In this chapter, we will explore the various benefits of nuts, their role in weight loss, and delve into the unique qualities of each type.

Nutritional Powerhouses

Nuts are nature's nutritional powerhouses, offering a wide array of health benefits. They are an excellent source of heart-healthy monounsaturated and polyunsaturated fats, known to reduce LDL cholesterol levels and promote cardiovascular health. The combination of healthy fats, protein, and fiber in nuts helps create a feeling of fullness, making them a satisfying and satiating snack that curbs hunger and reduces the urge to overeat.

Additionally, nuts are packed with essential vitamins and minerals, including vitamin E, magnesium, potassium, and antioxidants like selenium. These nutrients play crucial roles in various bodily functions, such as supporting the immune system, maintaining bone health, and protecting the body from oxidative stress.

Promoting Weight Loss

Contrary to their high-calorie content, studies have shown that including nuts in a weight loss diet can be beneficial. The combination of healthy fats, protein, and fiber in nuts helps regulate appetite and can contribute to reduced calorie intake throughout the day. Moreover, the slow digestion of nuts can lead to increased energy expenditure and a boost in metabolism.

It's important to note that while nuts are a nutritious addition to a weight loss plan, portion control is essential. Since nuts are calorie-dense, it's easy to consume large quantities without realizing the calorie intake. A small handful of nuts is a satisfying and nutrient-rich snack that can help you stay on track with your weight loss goals.

Various Nuts and Their Benefits:

1. Almonds

Almonds are one of the most popular and widely consumed nuts worldwide. Almonds stand out as an excellent source of essential nutrients, including vitamin E, magnesium, and calcium. Vitamin E, a potent antioxidant present in almonds, plays a vital role in shielding our cells from potential damage caused by free radicals. This protective function helps promote overall health and well-being. Almonds' high fiber content supports digestive health, and their monounsaturated fats have been linked to improved heart health. Additionally, the combination of protein and healthy fats in almonds helps stabilize blood sugar levels, reducing the risk of unhealthy food cravings.

2. Walnuts

Walnuts stand out as a unique nut due to their high content of alpha-linolenic acid (ALA), a type of omega-3 fatty acid. These heart-healthy fats have anti-inflammatory properties and support brain health. Walnuts are also rich in antioxidants, including ellagic acid and polyphenols, which help combat oxidative stress and inflammation in the body. Studies have shown that incorporating walnuts into the diet may have beneficial effects on heart health, brain function, and even weight management.

3. Cashews

Cashews have a buttery and creamy taste, making them a versatile nut used in both savory and sweet dishes. They are a good source of zinc, iron, and selenium. Selenium is an essential mineral that plays a key role in antioxidant defense systems, supporting the body's ability to fight oxidative damage. Cashews are lower in fat compared to other nuts, but the majority of their fat content is heart-healthy monounsaturated fat. They are also rich in plant-based protein, making them a great option for vegetarians and vegans.

4. Pistachios

Pistachios are not only delicious but also fun to eat, thanks to their in-shell nature. The act of shelling pistachios can help with portion control, as it slows down eating and gives the brain more time to register fullness. Pistachios are a good source of protein, fiber, and antioxidants, including lutein and zeaxanthin, which are beneficial for eye health. Moreover, they are lower in calories compared to some other nuts, making them an ideal choice for those mindful of their calorie intake.

5. Brazil Nuts

Brazil nuts are a rich source of selenium, an essential mineral that plays a key role in thyroid function and supports the immune system. Just a couple of Brazil nuts can provide your daily recommended intake of selenium. However, due to their high selenium content, it's essential not to over consume them. Selenium is necessary for the proper functioning of the thyroid gland, which plays a crucial role in regulating metabolism and weight management.

6. Hazelnuts

Hazelnuts are known for their delightful flavor and are commonly used in spreads like Nutella. They are a good source of vitamin E, which supports skin health and acts as an antioxidant to protect cells from damage. Hazelnuts also contain healthy fats that contribute to heart health. Furthermore, hazelnuts contain dietary fiber, which supports digestive health and helps in maintaining regular bowel movements.

7. Pecans

Pecans have a rich, buttery taste and are a favorite in desserts and baked goods. They are a good source of manganese and copper, essential minerals that support various enzymatic processes in the body. Manganese plays a vital role in energy metabolism and helps maintain healthy bones, while copper supports iron absorption and aids in the formation of collagen and connective tissues. Pecans also contain antioxidants, including flavonoids and phenolic compounds, which help combat oxidative stress and inflammation.

Incorporating Nuts into Your Diet

Nuts can be enjoyed in various ways, from snacking on a handful of raw nuts to adding them to salads, yogurt, oatmeal, and smoothies. You can also incorporate nuts into your baking and cooking to add texture and flavor to dishes. Just remember to practice portion control, as even though nuts are healthy, excessive consumption can lead to excess calorie intake.

A Word of Caution

While nuts offer an array of health benefits, some individuals may have allergies to certain types of nuts. If you are allergic to nuts, it's crucial to avoid them completely to prevent severe allergic reactions. Additionally, if you have any specific dietary restrictions or medical conditions, it's advisable to consult with a healthcare professional or a registered dietitian before adding nuts to your diet.

Nuts are a delightful and nutritious addition to any diet, and their unique combination of healthy fats, protein, fiber, vitamins, and minerals make them a valuable aid in weight loss. From almonds to pecans, each nut brings its own set of health benefits to the table. By incorporating a variety of nuts into your diet and practicing portion control, you can savor the delectable flavors and harness the weight loss potential of these tiny wonders.

With their scrumptious taste, versatile uses, and impressive nutrient profile, nuts are a must-have snack for anyone seeking to achieve weight loss goals while still savoring the pleasures of delicious and wholesome foods. Remember, moderation is key, and by making nuts a part of your balanced diet, you'll reap their numerous health benefits and find joy in nourishing your body with nature's little nutritional gems.

Juices

In the quest for a balanced and healthy diet, juices have emerged as delightful elixirs, offering both taste and nutrition. Replacing sugary drinks with natural, fresh fruit and vegetable juices can be a wise choice for those seeking to achieve weight loss goals. Let's delve into the world of juices and explore their benefits, especially when it comes to weight management.

The Appeal of Juices

Juices are undeniably enticing and refreshing beverages, packed with the goodness of fruits and vegetables. They offer a wide range of flavors, from tangy and zesty to sweet and soothing, making them a treat for the taste buds. Apart from their deliciousness, juices provide essential vitamins, minerals, and antioxidants that support overall well-being.

Juices for Weight Loss

Juices can play a beneficial role in a weight loss diet, particularly when consumed mindfully. They are often lower in calories compared to sugary sodas and other processed beverages, making them a healthier option. The key to using juices for weight loss lies in moderation and selecting ingredients wisely. Opt for juices that are made from fresh, whole fruits and vegetables without added sugars or artificial additives.

1. Pomegranate Juice

Pomegranate juice is a treasure trove of antioxidants, especially polyphenols and anthocyanins, which are known for their anti-inflammatory properties. These compounds help protect cells from damage, contribute to heart health, and support a healthy immune system. Pomegranate juice's natural sweetness adds a delightful twist to any juice blend.

2. Pineapple Juice

Pineapple juice is a tropical delight, offering a burst of tropical flavor with a touch of tanginess. It is an excellent source of vitamin C, which supports a robust immune system and aids in collagen production for healthy skin. Pineapple juice is also known for its bromelain content, an enzyme that aids digestion and reduces inflammation.

3. Cranberry Juice

Cranberry juice is celebrated for its potential to support urinary tract health due to its high content of proanthocyanidins, which help prevent harmful bacteria from adhering to the urinary tract lining. This juice can be slightly tart but is incredibly refreshing and offers a unique flavor profile.

4. Apple Juice

Apple juice is a classic favorite, loved for its sweet and crisp taste. The fiber content in apple juice aids in digestion and supports gut health. When making or buying apple juice, it's best to choose varieties with no added sugars or preservatives.

5. Watermelon Juice

Watermelon juice is a true summer delight, offering a refreshing and hydrating experience. It is a great source of hydration, as watermelon contains over 90% water. Watermelon also provides vitamins A and C, as well as lycopene, a powerful antioxidant that may have heart health benefits.

6. Carrot Juice

Carrot juice is a nutritious elixir that packs a punch of beta-carotene, a precursor to vitamin A. The natural sweetness of carrots makes this juice appealing and enjoyable.

7. Pear Juice

Pear juice is both smooth and subtly sweet, making it an excellent choice for juicing. Pears are a good source of dietary fiber, which aids in digestion and helps maintain a healthy gut. They also contain potassium, vitamin C, and antioxidants that promote overall well-being.

8. Lemon Juice

Lemon juice is a zesty addition to any juice blend, offering a tangy and refreshing flavor. Lemons are rich in vitamin C, which supports immune health and acts as an antioxidant. Lemon juice can add brightness and flavor to vegetable-based juices, enhancing their taste and appeal.

9. Cucumber Juice

Cucumber juice is incredibly hydrating and offers a subtle, cooling taste. Cucumbers are low in calories and rich in water, making them an excellent choice for weight loss. Additionally, cucumber juice contains silica, a compound that supports healthy skin and connective tissues.

10. Grape Juice

Grape juice, especially when made from dark-colored grapes, contains powerful antioxidants like resveratrol, which has been linked to various health benefits, including heart health. The natural sweetness of grape juice makes it a delightful treat without the need for added sugars.

11. Orange Juice

Orange juice is a classic and popular juice known for its refreshing taste and abundant vitamin C content. This citrus delight is packed with nutrients, including potassium, folate, and thiamine. Vitamin C is an essential antioxidant that boosts the immune system, supports collagen production for healthy skin, and aids in the absorption of iron. The natural sweetness of oranges makes their juice a delightful and nourishing addition to any juice blend.

Incorporating Juices

Juices can be enjoyed on their own as a refreshing beverage, or they can be combined to create delicious and nutritious blends. The versatility of juices allows for endless possibilities to suit your taste preferences and nutritional needs. Additionally, homemade juices offer the advantage of knowing exactly what ingredients are used, ensuring freshness and quality.

Choosing Wisely

When purchasing store-bought juices, opt for 100% pure fruit juice without added sugars, artificial flavors, or preservatives. It's best to read the labels and choose products with minimal or no additives. Making your own juices from fresh fruits and vegetables is the healthiest option, allowing you to control the quality and tailor the flavors to your liking.

Juices are not only a delightful indulgence but also a nourishing addition to a healthy diet. From the exotic flavors of pomegranate and pineapple to the classic appeal of apple and orange, each juice brings its unique set of nutrients and taste to the table. By incorporating a variety of fresh juices into your diet, you can relish the natural sweetness and reap the benefits of these liquid wonders. Whether it's a refreshing start to your day or a mid-afternoon pick-me-up, let the goodness of juices fuel your journey to a healthier and more vibrant life.

Cooking Oils, Butter, and Margarine

In the heart of every kitchen lies a diverse array of cooking oils, butter, and margarine, each playing a crucial role in enhancing flavors and textures of our favorite dishes. However, the choices we make in regards to these cooking fats can significantly impact our overall health. Understanding the importance of using healthy oils and making mindful selections of butter and margarine is vital for maintaining a balanced and nourishing diet. Let's embark on a journey through the world of cooking oils, butter, and margarine to uncover the key considerations and suggestions for creating a healthier and more vibrant kitchen.

The Importance of Using Healthy Oils

Cooking oils are the building blocks of culinary creations, offering a wealth of flavors and nutritional benefits. The right oil can elevate the taste of dishes while contributing to the overall health of our bodies. The focus should be on choosing cooking oils that are rich in unsaturated fats, such as monounsaturated and polyunsaturated fats, while minimizing the intake of saturated and trans fats. Unsaturated fats have been linked to various health benefits, including promoting heart health, reducing inflammation, and improving cholesterol levels.

Olive Oil - The Mediterranean Elixir

Olive oil, especially extra virgin olive oil, is hailed as one of the healthiest choices for cooking. Obtained directly from olives without any heat or chemicals, extra virgin olive oil retains its full flavor and nutritional value. It is rich in monounsaturated fats, particularly oleic acid, which has been linked to reduced heart disease risk. The oil is also packed with antioxidants like polyphenols, providing anti-inflammatory properties and protection against oxidative stress. For cooking, it is best used for low to medium heat methods to preserve its delicate flavors and nutrients.

Avocado Oil

The Green Gold: Avocado oil is another gem in the world of healthy cooking fats. Rich in monounsaturated fats, it shares similar heart-healthy benefits with olive oil. Its mild flavor and high smoke point make it versatile for sautéing, grilling, and roasting. Avocado oil is also abundant in vitamin E and beneficial plant compounds, making it a valuable addition to both savory and sweet dishes.

Coconut Oil

A Controversial Choice: Coconut oil has garnered attention in recent years due to its unique composition of medium-chain triglycerides (MCTs). While some studies suggest potential benefits, it is important to note that coconut oil contains a high proportion of saturated fats. Thus, it's best to use coconut oil in moderation and balance it with healthier cooking oils.

Sunflower Oil

Sunflower oil comes in different types, including high-oleic and mid-oleic varieties. High-oleic sunflower oil has a higher monounsaturated fat content and a longer shelf life. It is suitable for higher-temperature cooking like frying and roasting, while the mid-oleic type serves general cooking purposes. Sunflower oil is a good source of vitamin E and low in saturated fats, making it a healthier option compared to oils with higher saturated fat content.

Canola Oil

A Neutral All-Rounder: Canola oil is known for its light flavor and balanced fatty acid profile. Low in saturated fats and rich in monounsaturated fats, canola oil is considered heart-healthy. Its neutral taste makes it suitable for various cooking methods, from sautéing to baking, and it can improve cholesterol levels when used as part of a balanced diet.

The Role of Butter and Margarine

Butter and margarine, often used interchangeably in recipes, are both cherished for their rich flavors. However, it's essential to be mindful of their respective nutritional profiles.

Butter

Butter is a natural fat sourced from dairy and provides a distinctive richness to dishes. When choosing butter, opting for varieties sourced from grass-fed cows is beneficial, as they contain higher levels of essential nutrients like omega-3 fatty acids and antioxidants. Unsalted butter allows for better control over sodium intake. While butter can be part of a balanced diet, it is calorie-dense and contains saturated fats, so moderation is key.

Margarine

Traditional margarine, often containing trans fats, is not a health-conscious choice. However, trans fat-free margarine made from non-hydrogenated vegetable oils offers a healthier alternative. Look for margarines low in saturated fats and free from harmful trans fats. It can be a good option for spreading on bread or toast when used in moderation.

Incorporating Healthy Fats Into Your Kitchen

Incorporating a variety of healthy cooking oils, butter, and margarine into your kitchen repertoire allows for diverse flavors and nutritional benefits. When selecting cooking oils, consider their smoke points, nutritional profiles, and suitability for various cooking methods. Using a combination of oils, such as olive oil for low to medium heat cooking and sunflower or canola oil for high-heat cooking, ensures that you maximize the health benefits of each oil while elevating the taste of your dishes.

In the quest for a healthier kitchen and a balanced diet, the choices we make regarding cooking oils, butter, and margarine matter. By embracing the goodness of olive oil, avocado oil, and other healthy cooking oils, we not only enrich the flavors of our dishes but also nourish our bodies with essential nutrients and health benefits. Incorporating these healthier fats into our culinary adventures, we can create delicious and nutritious meals that contribute to our overall well-being. So, let's embark on a culinary journey filled with mindful choices and delightful flavors, making every dish a celebration of taste and health.

Don't Eat These Foods

In the pursuit of a healthier lifestyle and successful weight loss, being mindful of the foods we consume is crucial. Some commonly eaten foods can undermine our efforts and contribute to obesity and health issues. In this chapter, we'll explore a range of unhealthy foods to avoid to promote better well-being and achieve our weight loss goals.

Cheese with High Fat

Cheese, while delicious, can be high in saturated fats and calories. Consuming excessive amounts of high-fat cheese can lead to weight gain and an increased risk of heart disease.

Bacon

This savory and crispy treat is rich in unhealthy fats and sodium, making it an unfavorable choice for weight loss.

BBQ Sauce

Many BBQ sauces are packed with added sugars and high in calories.

Belgian Waffle

Belgian waffles are often loaded with refined flour, sugar, and topped with unhealthy syrups, leading to a high-calorie indulgence.

Bouillon Cube

These cubes contain high levels of sodium, which can contribute to water retention and bloating.

Cake

Celebration cakes are typically high in added sugars and unhealthy fats, making them a calorie-dense treat.

Candy

Candies are mostly made of sugars and offer little to no nutritional value, leading to empty calories.

Canned Soup

Many canned soups contain excessive sodium and preservatives, which are not conducive to a healthy diet.

Charred Meat

Grilling meat at high temperatures can produce harmful compounds that may contribute to health issues.

Cheesecake

This delectable dessert combines the drawbacks of cake with high-fat cream cheese, adding extra calories.

Chewing Gum

While sugar-free gum is better, chewing gum may lead to increased hunger and overeating.

Chips

Potato chips and other fried snacks are high in unhealthy fats and often laden with sodium.

Coffee Creamer

Commercial coffee creamers can contain added sugars and unhealthy fats.

Cookies

Cookies, especially store-bought varieties, are high in sugars, unhealthy fats, and empty calories.

Croissants

These flaky pastries are high in refined flour and unhealthy fats, contributing to weight gain.

Doughnuts

Doughnuts are deep-fried and laden with sugars and unhealthy fats.

Dried Fruit Snack

Dried fruits can be concentrated sources of sugars and calories when consumed in large quantities.

Fast Food (e.g., burgers, fries, fried chicken)

Fast food items are often high in unhealthy fats, sodium, and calories, leading to weight gain and adverse health effects.

Fettuccine Alfredo

This creamy pasta dish is rich in calories, saturated fats, and unhealthy cheeses.

Fish and Chips

The classic fish and chips combo is fried, leading to high unhealthy fat content.

Flavored Rice

Pre-packaged flavored rice often contains added sugars, sodium, and preservatives.

French Toast

This breakfast favorite is made with refined bread and soaked in sweet syrups, contributing to excessive calorie intake.

Frosting

Frostings are high in sugars and unhealthy fats, making them a weight loss hindrance.

Fried Chicken

Fried chicken is coated in unhealthy breading and high in saturated fats.

Fried Mozzarella Sticks

These deep-fried cheese sticks provide little nutritional value and are high in unhealthy fats.

Frozen Pie

Store-bought frozen pies often contain high levels of added sugars and unhealthy fats.

Frozen Pizza

Frozen pizzas are typically high in calories, unhealthy fats, and sodium.

Fruit Cocktail (high in added sugars)

Canned fruit cocktails may contain added sugars, negating the nutritional benefits of natural fruits.

Fruit Juice (high in added sugars)

Many fruit juices are concentrated sources of sugars without the beneficial fiber found in whole fruits.

Granola Bar (often high in sugar and calories)

Some granola bars can be calorie-dense and loaded with added sugars.

Greasy Burgers

Greasy burgers are high in unhealthy fats, sodium, and empty calories.

Greasy Pizza

Pizza topped with excessive cheese and unhealthy meats can be high in calories and saturated fats.

Hot Dog

Hot dogs are processed meats, often high in sodium and unhealthy additives.

Ketchup (high in added sugars)

Many commercial ketchups contain high amounts of added sugars, which can hinder weight loss efforts.

Margarine

Some margarines may contain unhealthy trans fats, making them an undesirable choice.

Mayonnaise

Mayonnaise is high in unhealthy fats and calories and should be used sparingly.

Meatloaf (depending on preparation)

Meatloaf made with fatty meats or excessive additives can be detrimental to weight loss efforts.

Nachos

Loaded with cheese, sour cream, and processed toppings, nachos are a high-calorie indulgence.

Onion Ring

Onion rings are deep-fried, adding unhealthy fats and calories.

Pancake Syrup (high in added sugars)

Commercial pancake syrups are often high in added sugars and artificial flavors.

Pickle (often high in sodium)

Pickles may contain excessive sodium, contributing to water retention.

Pizza (especially with extra cheese and toppings)

Pizzas loaded with unhealthy toppings can be calorie-dense and high in unhealthy fats.

Processed Meat (e.g., sausages, deli meats)

Processed meats are often high in sodium, preservatives, and unhealthy fats.

Protein Bar (some may be high in sugars and calories)

Some protein bars can be more like candy bars, with high sugars and unhealthy additives.

Refried Beans (if high in fat and sodium)

Refried beans can be calorie-dense when cooked with unhealthy fats.

Salad Dressing (some high-calorie and high-fat options)

Creamy salad dressings can be high in unhealthy fats and calories.

Sausage (high in fat and sodium)

Sausages are processed meats with high levels of unhealthy fats and sodium.

Sauces with added sugars and unhealthy fats

Some sauces, like certain barbecue and sweet chili sauces, may contain added sugars and unhealthy fats.

Sugary Cereal

Sweetened cereals are high in added sugars and provide little nutritional value.

Taco Bowl (if high in unhealthy ingredients)

Taco bowls loaded with unhealthy toppings and sauces can be high in calories.

Tiramisu (high in sugar and fat)

This indulgent dessert is rich in sugars and unhealthy fats.

Veggie Burger (depending on preparation and ingredients)

Some veggie burgers may be highly processed and contain unhealthy additives.

Wheat Bread (highly processed)

Certain wheat bread varieties may contain added sugars and unhealthy additives.

White Sugar (added sugar in various foods)

White sugar is a common source of empty calories and contributes to weight gain.

Noodle Soup (if high in sodium and unhealthy fats)

Certain instant noodle soups can be high in sodium and unhealthy fats.

By avoiding these unhealthy foods and making mindful choices in our diet, we can work towards a healthier lifestyle and achieve our weight loss goals more effectively. Prioritizing whole, unprocessed foods and incorporating balanced meals will set us on the path to improved well-being and long-term health. Remember, moderation is key, and a balanced approach to nutrition is essential for sustainable weight management.

Don't Drink These Drinks and Beverages

In the quest for a healthier lifestyle and successful weight loss, it is essential to pay close attention to the beverages we consume. The impact of our drink choices on our overall health and weight management cannot be underestimated. Many commonly consumed drinks and beverages are laden with added sugars and empty calories, which can lead to weight gain and various health issues. Let's explore in detail the various types of drinks to avoid and the reasons behind their harmful effects on our bodies.

1. Sweetened Teas

Tea is a popular beverage enjoyed by people worldwide for its comforting and refreshing qualities. However, sweetened teas are a major culprit when it comes to hidden added sugars. These sugary concoctions can be found in a variety of flavors, including black tea, green tea, Earl Grey, jasmine, chai, and more. The excessive sugar content in sweetened teas can contribute to weight gain and negatively impact our blood sugar levels. Additionally, the habit of consuming sweetened teas may contribute to a preference for overly sweet tastes, making it challenging to enjoy natural flavors from whole foods.

2. Sugary Sodas

Regular soda drinks, such as cola, lemon-lime, and other carbonated beverages, are among the most significant sources of added sugars in the modern diet. These fizzy drinks are not only calorie-dense but also devoid of essential nutrients. Regularly consuming sugary sodas can have detrimental effects on your health. These beverages are high in added sugars, which can contribute to weight gain and an increased risk of chronic conditions such as type 2 diabetes and heart disease. Additionally, the high sugar content in sodas can also lead to tooth decay, causing further harm to your overall well-being. It is essential to be mindful of your soda intake and consider healthier alternatives to support your overall health and weight management goals. Studies have linked high soda intake to insulin resistance and metabolic disturbances, making it a harmful choice for those seeking to manage their weight and improve their overall health.

3. Fruit Juices with Added Sugars

Fruit juices may appear healthy at first glance due to their association with natural fruits. However, many commercially available fruit juices are heavily processed and contain added sugars. The natural sugars present in whole fruits are accompanied by beneficial fiber, which helps slow down sugar absorption and provides a sense of fullness. When fruit juices are stripped of fiber and loaded with extra sugars, they become calorie-dense and can lead to spikes in blood sugar levels. Consuming fruit juices with added sugars can hinder weight loss efforts and contribute to fluctuations in energy levels.

4. Sweetened Coffee Drinks

Coffee, a beloved morning beverage for many, can quickly turn into a calorie bomb when transformed into sweetened coffee drinks like flavored lattes and mochas. These popular creations often contain high amounts of sugar and unhealthy syrups, which not only add unnecessary calories but may also lead to energy crashes and cravings for more sugary treats. It's essential to be mindful of the ingredients in coffee drinks and choose simpler, less sweetened options to avoid sabotaging weight loss goals.

5. Energy Drinks

Marketed as boosters for increased energy and mental alertness, energy drinks are notorious for their high sugar and caffeine content. These beverages may provide a temporary surge of energy but are not a sustainable solution for combatting fatigue. The excess sugar and caffeine in energy drinks can lead to jitteriness, insomnia, and even dependency on these drinks to stay awake. Moreover, the high calorie content of energy drinks can contribute to weight gain if consumed frequently.

6. Sports Drinks and Vitamin Waters

Often advertised as essential for hydration and replenishing electrolytes, sports drinks and vitamin waters are commonly perceived as healthy options. However, many of these beverages are loaded with added sugars, undermining their potential benefits. Unless you engage in intense physical activity that requires specific electrolyte replenishment, these sugary beverages are unnecessary. Opting for plain water or natural electrolyte sources, such as coconut water, is a better choice for overall health and weight management.

7. Flavored Milk and Milkshakes

Milk, an excellent source of essential nutrients like calcium and protein, can lose its health benefits when transformed into flavored milk or milkshakes loaded with added sugars. These sweetened dairy beverages are calorie-dense and can contribute to unhealthy weight gain if consumed regularly. Instead of reaching for pre-sweetened options, opt for unsweetened milk and flavor it with natural ingredients like vanilla extract or unsweetened cocoa powder for a healthier and more flavorful alternative.

8. Alcoholic Beverages

Alcoholic drinks, such as beer, cocktails, and sweet wines, are not only high in empty calories but can also have a negative impact on our weight and overall health. Alcoholic beverages provide calories without offering any essential nutrients, leading to a phenomenon known as "empty calories." Moreover, excessive alcohol consumption can hinder weight loss efforts as our bodies prioritize metabolizing alcohol over burning fat for energy. Additionally, alcohol can impair judgment and lead to poor food choices, making it more likely to indulge in unhealthy foods when under the influence.

9. Sweetened Plant-based Milks

Plant-based milk alternatives, such as almond milk, soy milk, and coconut milk, have gained popularity as dairy alternatives. While unsweetened versions of these plant-based milks can be healthy choices, sweetened varieties often contain added sugars. Always opt for unsweetened plant-based milks to avoid unnecessary sugar intake and enjoy the natural flavors of these alternatives.

10. Sweetened Iced Tea

Iced tea, a refreshing option on hot days, can become problematic when sweetened with added sugars. Commercially prepared sweetened iced tea can be loaded with sugar, contributing to excessive calorie intake and potential weight gain. Making iced tea at home and sweetening it with natural sweeteners like honey or a small amount of fruit juice can be a healthier alternative.

Avoiding these unhealthy drinks and beverages can have a significant positive impact on your health and weight loss journey. Instead, prioritize hydration with plain water, herbal teas without added sugars, or plain coffee or tea without sweeteners. By making mindful beverage choices, you can support your weight loss goals and enhance your overall well-being. Remember that small changes in your daily drink choices can lead to significant improvements in your health and quality of life.

Healthy Lifestyle

A healthy lifestyle is a key determinant of overall well-being and plays a pivotal role in achieving and maintaining weight loss goals. Embracing a holistic approach to health encompasses various aspects of life that contribute to physical, mental, and emotional harmony. In this chapter, we will delve into the essential components of a healthy lifestyle, their benefits, and their significance for achieving optimal health and weight management.

Sleep is a fundamental pillar of good health, and its significance cannot be overstated. Quality sleep is essential for the body's recovery and rejuvenation processes, which promote physical and mental health. During sleep, the body repairs tissues, consolidates memories, and regulates hormones, including those involved in appetite and metabolism. Lack of sufficient sleep can lead to hormonal imbalances, increased cravings for unhealthy foods, and reduced motivation for physical activity, making it harder to maintain a healthy weight. To embrace a healthy lifestyle, prioritize sleep and aim for 7-9 hours of restful sleep each night.

Furthermore, ample rest enhances cognitive function and emotional stability, helping you make better decisions regarding your diet and physical activities. Studies have shown that individuals who don't get enough sleep are more likely to consume high-calorie and unhealthy foods while feeling less inclined to engage in exercise.

Effective time management is crucial for achieving a healthy lifestyle. When you manage your time wisely, you can strike a balance between work, personal life, and healthy habits. Setting clear goals and priorities helps you allocate time to essential activities, such as cooking nutritious meals, exercising, and engaging in self-care practices. Time management also reduces stress and prevents burnout, as you are better equipped to handle tasks efficiently and with a sense of purpose.

By planning your days with care, you create an environment that encourages healthy choices. Allocating time for meal preparation, for instance, ensures that you have access to nourishing and well-balanced meals. Regular exercise becomes a part of your routine, making it less likely for you to skip workouts due to time constraints. Effective time management empowers you to optimize your schedule and align it with your health and wellness objectives.

Proper planning is instrumental in maintaining a healthy lifestyle. By scheduling your daily, weekly, and monthly activities in advance, you can avoid last-minute rushes and create a structured routine that supports your health goals. Planning meals ahead of time allows you to make healthier food choices and avoid impulsive decisions that may lead to consuming unhealthy options. Additionally, scheduling regular exercise sessions ensures that physical activity becomes a consistent part of your routine.

The act of planning fosters mindfulness, enabling you to be conscious of your decisions and actions. This mindfulness extends to your dietary choices, encouraging you to select nutrient-dense and wholesome foods. When you plan your meals, you are less likely to opt for fast-food or processed snacks. Similarly, scheduling exercise sessions motivates you to commit to regular physical activity, which is crucial for weight loss and maintaining a healthy body composition.

The company we keep greatly influences our mindset and lifestyle choices. Being in the company of positive and sincere individuals who prioritize their health and well-being can be motivating and encouraging. Positive social interactions promote mental and emotional well-being, reducing stress and promoting a positive outlook on life. Surround yourself with people who share similar health goals, as this creates a supportive environment that fosters healthy habits and mutual encouragement.

Social support is a powerful tool in your weight loss journey. Engaging with like-minded individuals who are also pursuing a healthy lifestyle can provide motivation, accountability, and encouragement. Whether it's joining a fitness class, a weight loss support group, or simply spending time with friends who share your commitment to health, being surrounded by positive influences can significantly impact your success in achieving and maintaining a healthy weight.

In the digital age, smartphones, tablets, and other electronic devices have become an integral part of daily life. However, excessive screen time can hinder a healthy lifestyle by taking away valuable time that could be spent on activities that promote well-being. Constantly surfing the internet, chatting online, or engaging in social media can lead to sedentary behaviors and mindless eating. Limiting screen time allows you to be more present and mindful, engaging in physical activities and connecting with others face-to-face.

Excessive screen time is associated with a sedentary lifestyle, which can negatively impact weight management. People often consume high-calorie snacks mindlessly while engaging with screens, contributing to weight gain. By reducing screen time, you create opportunities to be physically active, engage in mindful eating, and foster real-life connections. Go for a walk, participate in outdoor activities, or spend quality time with loved ones without the distraction of screens.

A healthy lifestyle is not a quick fix but rather a lifelong journey of nurturing your body, mind, and spirit. By committing to principles like prioritizing restful sleep, effective time management, and positive social connections, you can achieve lasting health, happiness, and balance in your life. Embrace the importance of a healthy lifestyle and let it guide you towards overall well-being and successful weight management. Remember, it's not just about reaching your weight loss goals; it's about cultivating a fulfilling and vibrant life through positive habits and conscious choices. With determination and dedication, you can make a remarkable difference in your life and experience the joy of a truly healthy lifestyle.

In conclusion, adopting a healthy lifestyle is essential for achieving and maintaining weight loss goals while enhancing overall well-being. Each component of a healthy lifestyle, from sufficient sleep to time management, social connections, and reducing screen time, contributes to a harmonious and fulfilling existence. By nurturing your body, mind, and spirit, you create a strong foundation for sustained health and happiness. Remember, healthy living is not a destination but a lifelong journey of growth, self-discovery, and positive transformation. As you embrace a healthy lifestyle, you empower yourself to lead a life that is vibrant, energetic, and full of vitality. Your commitment to health will reward you with abundant rewards, including a body that feels strong, a mind that is sharp, and a heart that is content.

Healthy Activities, Sports, Hobbies

Engaging in healthy activities, sports, and hobbies plays a crucial role in achieving your weight loss goals while promoting overall well-being. Incorporating enjoyable and sustainable activities into your daily routine not only aids in shedding unwanted pounds but also enhances your physical fitness, mental health, and overall quality of life. In this chapter, we will explore the significance of sports, outdoor activities, and hobbies in supporting your journey towards a healthier and happier self.

Sports

Participating in sports provides a dynamic and enjoyable way to stay active and burn calories. Whether it's team sports like soccer, basketball, or individual sports like tennis, swimming, or cycling, sports offer numerous benefits for weight loss and overall fitness. Playing sports involves continuous movement, which helps boost your metabolism and accelerates fat burning. Additionally, sports are a great way to improve your cardiovascular health, muscular strength, and coordination.

Beyond the physical advantages, sports also promote social interactions and teamwork, fostering a sense of camaraderie and support. Being part of a sports team can create a strong support system, encouraging you to stay committed to your fitness goals. Moreover, the competitive nature of sports can fuel your motivation and determination to excel, contributing to better performance and greater calorie expenditure.

To get the most out of sports as part of your weight loss journey, choose activities that you genuinely enjoy and find exciting. When you are passionate about the sport you engage in, you are more likely to remain consistent and dedicated in the long term. Whether it's playing casual games with friends or joining organized leagues, sports offer an engaging and rewarding way to achieve your fitness goals while having fun.

Outdoor Activities

Spending time outdoors and engaging in physical activities amidst nature provides a refreshing and rejuvenating experience. Outdoor activities such as hiking, cycling, jogging, or simply taking a brisk walk in the park can significantly contribute to weight loss and overall well-being. The natural surroundings not only inspire a sense of tranquility but also motivate you to be more active.

Outdoor activities offer a break from the monotony of indoor exercises, allowing you to breathe in fresh air and soak in the beauty of nature. Such activities engage various muscle groups and elevate your heart rate, leading to increased calorie burn and improved cardiovascular health. Additionally, exposure to natural sunlight helps regulate your circadian rhythm, improving sleep quality and supporting your weight loss efforts.

Engaging in outdoor hobbies like gardening can be especially beneficial. Gardening involves various physical activities such as digging, planting, weeding, and watering, providing a moderate-intensity workout that enhances flexibility, strength, and endurance. Beyond the physical benefits, gardening also promotes mental well-being, reduces stress, and fosters a connection with nature.

Hobbies

Incorporating hobbies into your daily routine not only brings joy and fulfillment but also contributes to a healthy lifestyle. Hobbies can range from artistic pursuits like painting, drawing, or playing a musical instrument to more physically engaging activities like dancing, martial arts, or yoga. Engaging in hobbies provides a sense of purpose and accomplishment, reducing stress and promoting mental well-being.

Certain hobbies, such as dancing or yoga, are not only enjoyable but also effective in burning calories and improving flexibility and balance. These activities also encourage mindfulness and body awareness, which can translate to better eating habits and more conscious food choices.

The key to incorporating hobbies into your weight loss journey is to allocate time for these activities regularly. Treat your hobbies as essential self-care practices that not only bring happiness but also contribute to your physical and mental health. By dedicating time to pursue your hobbies, you create a positive and balanced lifestyle that supports your weight loss goals.

Exploring new hobbies can also be an exciting way to discover activities that spark your interest and passion. Whether it's learning a new dance style, trying a martial arts class, taking up gardening, or exploring nature through bird-watching, experimenting with different hobbies keeps your fitness routine fresh and enjoyable.

Hobbies can also be a fantastic way to connect with others who share similar interests. Joining hobby groups, clubs, or classes provides an opportunity to socialize, make new friends, and foster a sense of belonging. This social support network can be invaluable in staying motivated and accountable on your weight loss journey.

Moreover, engaging in creative hobbies, such as painting, writing, or crafting, can serve as a form of emotional expression and stress relief. Expressing yourself through artistic pursuits allows you to channel your emotions and emotions positively, leading to better emotional well-being and a reduced risk of emotional eating.

Engaging in healthy activities, sports, and hobbies offers multifaceted benefits that go beyond weight loss. Sports provide an avenue for physical fitness, teamwork, and friendly competition, while outdoor activities reconnect you with nature and boost your cardiovascular health. Hobbies, on the other hand, foster creativity, reduce stress, and enhance mindfulness.

By choosing activities that you genuinely enjoy and align with your interests, you can cultivate a sustainable and enjoyable fitness routine. The key to long-term success lies in finding activities that bring you joy, motivating you to stay consistent and committed to your health and weight loss goals.

A healthy lifestyle is not solely about rigorous exercise routines; it encompasses a diverse array of activities that nourish your body, mind, and soul. Embrace the power of sports, outdoor adventures, and hobbies to create a vibrant and fulfilling life that supports your well-being and empowers you to achieve your weight loss aspirations.

Connecting with Nature's Rhythms

Nature operates on its own unique rhythm and cycle. Spending time outdoors exposes us to these natural patterns, such as the rising and setting of the sun, the changing seasons, and the ebb and flow of tides. Connecting with these rhythms can have a grounding effect on our bodies and minds.

Sunlight exposure during the day helps regulate our circadian rhythm, the internal clock that governs our sleep-wake cycle. A well-balanced circadian rhythm is essential for quality sleep, and proper rest is crucial for weight management. When our sleep patterns are disrupted due to irregular schedules or excessive exposure to artificial light at night, it can lead to imbalances in hunger-regulating hormones, potentially increasing appetite and cravings for unhealthy foods.

Furthermore, spending time in nature during the day exposes us to natural light, which has been shown to boost mood and energy levels. A positive mood can translate into better food choices and increased motivation to engage in physical activities, ultimately supporting weight loss efforts.

The Joy of Movement in Nature

One of the greatest benefits of spending time in nature is the joy of movement it encourages. Unlike indoor exercises that may feel monotonous and routine, outdoor activities offer a sense of adventure and exploration. Whether it's hiking through a lush forest, biking along scenic trails, or swimming in a pristine lake, physical activities in nature become exciting and invigorating experiences.

The joy of movement in nature also fosters a healthy relationship with exercise. Instead of viewing exercise as a chore or a means to an end, being active outdoors allows us to embrace movement as an enjoyable part of our daily lives. When we genuinely enjoy the activities we engage in, we are more likely to stick with them in the long term, making it easier to maintain a consistent exercise routine.

Nature as a Stress Buffer

Chronic stress can have a profound impact on our health and well-being, contributing to weight gain, inflammation, and an increased risk of chronic diseases. Nature acts as a natural stress buffer, providing a peaceful refuge from the demands and pressures of everyday life.

When we immerse ourselves in the beauty of nature, our bodies enter a state of relaxation and tranquility. The calming effects of natural environments activate the parasympathetic nervous system, which counters the stress response triggered by the sympathetic nervous system. This shift towards relaxation helps reduce cortisol levels and allows our bodies to recover from the negative effects of stress.

As we find solace in nature, we can release tension and worries, letting go of emotional burdens that may lead to emotional eating or overeating. Instead of turning to food as a coping mechanism, we can turn to the healing power of nature to find comfort and peace.

Family and Community Bonding in Nature

Spending time in nature also presents an excellent opportunity for family and community bonding. Engaging in outdoor activities together can strengthen relationships and create lasting memories. Whether it's going on a family hike, having a picnic in the park, or participating in community gardening, these shared experiences foster a sense of connection and belonging.

Family and community support are crucial for maintaining healthy habits and achieving weight loss goals. Having a support system that encourages and motivates us can make a significant difference in our health journey. Spending time in nature together not only promotes physical activity but also nurtures emotional bonds, creating a network of support that helps us stay on track with our wellness objectives.

Embracing Nature's Miracles

Nature has an abundance of healing wonders that can benefit our health and well-being. From natural herbs and plants with medicinal properties to the healing properties of natural bodies of water, the Earth offers a treasure trove of remedies for various ailments.

Exploring natural remedies can complement weight loss efforts by addressing underlying health issues or imbalances that may be hindering progress. Incorporating herbal teas, infusions, or using essential oils derived from plants can support overall well-being and encourage a more holistic approach to health.

Spending time in nature is a gift we can give ourselves, a gift that bestows numerous rewards for our physical, mental, and emotional health. The serenity, beauty, and therapeutic power of nature contribute to stress reduction, improved mood, and a heightened sense of well-being. As we embrace the tranquility of natural surroundings, we discover a profound connection with ourselves and the world around us.

Engaging in outdoor activities, sports, and hobbies in nature not only supports weight loss goals but also nurtures our mind, body, and spirit. The joy of movement in nature, coupled with the calming effects on our nervous system, helps us find balance, reduce stress, and make mindful choices that foster health and happiness.

In this fast-paced, technology-driven world, stepping into nature's embrace offers us a chance to pause, reflect, and appreciate the simple wonders of life. Let nature be your sanctuary, your escape from the noise and chaos, and your guide on the path to a healthier and more fulfilling life.

Embrace the healing power of nature and embark on a journey of well-being, knowing that the beauty and tranquility of nature are always waiting to welcome you home.

Final Word

As we arrive at the final chapter of "Easy Weight Loss Diet for Maximum Results," it is time to celebrate your journey of transformation and empowerment. Throughout this book, we have explored the essential components of a healthy lifestyle, delved into nutritious and delicious foods, and uncovered the significance of physical activity. Now, let's wrap up this incredible journey with a reflection on the key aspects and motivational insights that will inspire you to continue your path towards a healthier, happier you.

Your Health is Your Greatest Asset

As you embark on this journey towards a healthier life, always remember that your health is your most valuable asset. It impacts every aspect of your life, from your physical well-being to your emotional and mental state. Prioritizing your health not only enhances your quality of life but also empowers you to embrace every opportunity that comes your way. As you make positive changes in your diet and lifestyle, you are investing in a future filled with vitality, energy, and joy.

Consistency is Key

In any endeavor, consistency is the key to success. The same applies to your weight loss journey and the adoption of a healthy lifestyle. Consistency in your food choices, exercise routines, and self-care practices creates a strong foundation for lasting change. Remember that small, consistent actions add up over time, leading to significant and sustainable results. Be patient with yourself, celebrate your progress, and stay committed to your goals.

The Power of Mindful Eating

Mindful eating is a powerful practice that allows you to cultivate a deeper connection with your body and its nutritional needs. By paying attention to the tastes, textures, and sensations of each bite, you become more attuned to your hunger and satiety cues. This mindful approach to eating not only promotes healthier food choices but also prevents overeating and emotional eating. Savor your meals, embrace the joy of nourishing your body, and relish the simple pleasure of every culinary experience.

Embrace the Joy of Movement

Physical activity should never be a burden but a celebration of your body's capabilities. Find activities that bring you joy and excitement, whether it's dancing, hiking, yoga, or swimming. By engaging in activities you love, you are more likely to make exercise a regular part of your life. Let go of the idea that exercise is solely about burning calories; instead, focus on the joy, fulfillment, and stress-relief it brings. Movement is a gift to cherish, not a chore to endure.

Nurture Your Mental and Emotional Well-Being

A holistic approach to health includes nurturing your mental and emotional well-being. Make time for self-care practices that promote relaxation, reduce stress, and cultivate a sense of inner peace. Meditation, journaling, spending time in nature, and connecting with loved ones are powerful ways to nourish your soul. By caring for your mental health, you enhance your ability to cope with challenges, make better decisions, and maintain a positive outlook on life.

Redefine Success and Progress

In your pursuit of weight loss and a healthy lifestyle, redefine your definition of success and progress. Instead of solely focusing on the number on the scale, celebrate non-scale victories such as increased energy levels, improved sleep, enhanced mood, and increased confidence. Recognize that your worth is not tied to a specific weight or body shape, and embrace your uniqueness and individuality. Your journey is personal, and each step you take is a triumph in itself.

Build a Supportive Community

Surround yourself with a supportive community that shares your health goals and aspirations. Connect with family, friends, or online communities that encourage and uplift you. Share your challenges and triumphs, and draw strength from the collective support. Having a community of like-minded individuals by your side can make a significant difference in your motivation and commitment to a healthy lifestyle.

Embrace Resilience

Throughout your health journey, you may encounter setbacks and obstacles. Embrace resilience as you navigate these challenges and view them as opportunities for growth. Be kind to yourself and avoid self-criticism. Instead, use setbacks as stepping stones to learn, adapt, and move forward with even greater determination. Remember that every successful journey includes moments of struggle and triumph; your resilience will guide you through it all.

Cultivate Self-Compassion

Practicing self-compassion is paramount in maintaining a positive mindset and fostering a healthy relationship with yourself. Be gentle and understanding when facing difficulties or setbacks. Treat yourself with the same love and empathy you would offer to a dear friend. Acknowledge that you are on a journey of growth, and every step, no matter how small, is worthy of celebration.

Celebrate Your Victories

Amidst the challenges and hard work, remember to celebrate your victories. Celebrate not just the big milestones but also the small triumphs that come along the way. Acknowledge your efforts, the progress you've made, and the positive changes you've incorporated into your life. Celebrating your successes reinforces your motivation, reinforces positive behaviors, and builds confidence in your ability to achieve your goals.

Your Journey, Your Life, Your Adventure

As you conclude this book and continue your health journey, remember that this is your life and your adventure. Embrace each day with gratitude, curiosity, and excitement for the possibilities that lie ahead. Cherish the moments of transformation and growth, for they shape the person you are becoming. This journey is about more than just weight loss; it is about reclaiming your health, embracing your vitality, and living life to the fullest.

By prioritizing your health, nurturing your well-being, and celebrating the journey, you will unlock the potential within you to achieve greatness. The decision to prioritize your health is an act of self-love, and it will ripple into every aspect of your life.

As you embark on this new chapter of your life, take with you the knowledge, wisdom, and motivation gained from this book. Remember that you are not alone; you have the strength of countless individuals who have walked this path before you and emerged stronger and more empowered.

May your health journey be filled with joy, resilience, and profound transformations. Stay true to your purpose, cherish your progress, and continue to thrive in the pursuit of your dreams.